Obstetric Anesthesia

Editors

ONYI C. ONUOHA
ROBERT R. GAISER

ANESTHESIOLOGY CLINICS

www.anesthesiology.theclinics.com

Consulting Editor
LEE A. FLEISHER

March 2017 • Volume 35 • Number 1

ELSEVIER

1600 John F. Kennedy Boulevard • Suite 1800 • Philadelphia, Pennsylvania, 19103-2899

http://www.theclinics.com

ANESTHESIOLOGY CLINICS Volume 35, Number 1
March 2017 ISSN 1932-2275, ISBN-13: 978-0-323-50972-5

Editor: Katie Pfaff
Developmental Editor: Kristen Helm

Anesthesiology Clinics (ISSN 1932-2275) is published quarterly by Elsevier Inc., 360 Park Avenue South, New York, NY 10010-1710. Months of issue are March, June, September, and December. Periodicals postage paid at New York, NY and at additional mailing offices. Subscription prices are $100.00 per year (US student/resident), $333.00 per year (US individuals), $404.00 per year (Canadian individuals), $620.00 per year (US institutions), $783.00 per year (Canadian institutions), $225.00 per year (Canadian and foreign student/resident), $460.00 per year (foreign individuals), and $783.00 per year (foreign institutions). To receive student and resident rate, orders must be accompanied by name of affiliated institution, date of term, and the *signature* of program/residency coordinator on institutions letterhead. Orders will be billed at individual rate until proof of status is received. Foreign air speed delivery is included in all *Clinics'* subscription prices. All prices are subject to change without notice. POSTMASTER: Send address changes to *Anesthesiology Clinics,* Elsevier Health Sciences Division, Subscription Customer Service, 3251 Riverport Lane, Maryland Heights, MO 63043. Customer Service (orders, claims, online, change of address): Elsevier Health Sciences Division, Subscription Customer Service, 3251 Riverport Lane, Maryland Heights, MO 63043. **Tel:1-800-654-2452 (U.S. and Canada); 314-447-8871 (outside U.S. and Canada). Fax: 314-447-8029. E-mail: journalscustomerservice-usa@elsevier. com (for print support); journalsonlinesupport-usa@elsevier.com (for online support).**

Reprints. For copies of 100 or more of articles in this publication, please contact the Commercial Reprints Department, Elsevier Inc., 360 Park Avenue South, New York, NY 10010-1710. Tel.: 212-633-3874; Fax: 212-633-3820; E-mail: reprints@elsevier.com.

Anesthesiology Clinics, is also published in Spanish by McGraw-Hill Inter-americana Editores S. A., P.O. Box 5-237, 06500 Mexico D. F., Mexico.

Anesthesiology Clinics, is covered in *MEDLINE/PubMed (Index Medicus), Current Contents/Clinical Medicine, Excerpta Medica, ISI/BIOMED,* and *Chemical Abstracts.*

Contributors

CONSULTING EDITOR

LEE A. FLEISHER, MD, FACC
Robert D. Dripps Professor and Chair of Anesthesiology and Critical Care, Professor of Medicine, Perelman School of Medicine, University of Pennsylvania, Philadelphia, Pennsylvania

EDITORS

ONYI C. ONUOHA, MD, MPH
Assistant Professor of Clinical Anesthesiology, Department of Anesthesiology and Critical Care, Perelman School of Medicine, University of Pennsylvania, Philadelphia, Pennsylvania

ROBERT R. GAISER, MD
Professor and Chair, Department of Anesthesiology, University of Kentucky, Lexington, Kentucky

AUTHORS

CRISTIAN ARZOLA, MD, MSc
Department of Anesthesia and Pain Management, Mount Sinai Hospital, University of Toronto, Toronto, Ontario, Canada

EMILY J. BAIRD, MD, PhD
Assistant Program Director of Resident Education and Scholarship; Assistant Professor of Anesthesiology and Perioperative Medicine, Department of Anesthesiology and Perioperative Medicine, Oregon Health and Science University, Portland, Oregon

CURTIS L. BAYSINGER, MD
Professor, Department of Anesthesiology, Vanderbilt University Medical Center, Nashville, Tennessee

BRENDAN CARVALHO, MBBCh, FRCA
Professor, Department of Anesthesiology, Perioperative and Pain Medicine, Stanford University School of Medicine, Stanford, California

JOSE C.A. CARVALHO, MD, PhD, FANZCA, FRCPC
Departments of Anesthesia and Pain Management, and Obstetrics and Gynecology, Mount Sinai Hospital, University of Toronto, Toronto, Ontario, Canada

ANNEMARIA DE TINA, MD, FRCPC
Clinical Fellow, Obstetric Anesthesiology, Department of Anesthesiology, Perioperative and Pain Medicine, Brigham and Women's Hospital, Boston, Massachusetts

NERLYNE K. DHARIWAL, MD
Anesthesiology Resident, Department of Anesthesiology, Emory University, Atlanta, Georgia

ROBERT R. GAISER, MD
Professor and Chair, Department of Anesthesiology, University of Kentucky, Lexington, Kentucky

NATHANIEL HSU, MD
Department of Anesthesiology and Critical Care, Hospital of the University of Pennsylvania, Philadelphia, Pennsylvania

STEPHANIE LIM, MD
Assistant Clinical Professor, Division of Obstetric Anesthesia, Department of Anesthesia & Perioperative Care, University of California San Francisco School of Medicine, San Francisco, California

BRANDON M. LOPEZ, MD
Assistant Professor, Department of Anesthesiology, University of Florida College of Medicine, Gainesville, Florida

JENNIFER LUCERO, MD
Assistant Professor of Clinical Anesthesia and Associate Clinical Director of Obstetric Anesthesia, Division of Obstetric Anesthesia, Department of Anesthesia & Perioperative Care; Department of Obstetrics, Gynecology & Reproductive Sciences, University of California San Francisco School of Medicine, San Francisco, California

GRANT C. LYNDE, MD, MBA
Associate Professor, Chief of Practice and Process Improvement, Department of Anesthesiology, Emory University, Atlanta, Georgia

EMILY McQUAID-HANSON, MD
Instructor in Anesthesia, Departments of Anesthesia, Critical Care, and Pain Medicine, Harvard Medical School, Massachusetts General Hospital, Boston, Massachusetts

ONYI C. ONUOHA, MD, MPH
Assistant Professor of Clinical Anesthesiology, Department of Anesthesiology and Critical Care, Perelman School of Medicine, University of Pennsylvania, Philadelphia, Pennsylvania

ARVIND PALANISAMY, MD, FRCA
Assistant Professor of Anesthesia, Department of Anesthesiology, Perioperative and Pain Medicine, Brigham and Women's Hospital, Harvard Medical School, Boston, Massachusetts

MAY C.M. PIAN-SMITH, MD
Associate Professor, Director of Quality and Safety, Departments of Anesthesia, Critical Care, and Pain Medicine, Harvard Medical School, Massachusetts General Hospital, Boston, Massachusetts

MICHAEL G. RICHARDSON, MD
Associate Professor, Department of Anesthesiology, Vanderbilt University Medical Center, Nashville, Tennessee

CAITLIN DOOLEY SUTTON, MD
Fellow, Department of Anesthesiology, Perioperative and Pain Medicine, Stanford University School of Medicine, Stanford, California

CHIRAAG TALATI, MBBS, BSc (Hons), FRCA
Department of Anaesthesia, Homerton University Hospital NHS Foundation Trust, Homerton Row, London, United Kingdom

Contents

> Despite the traditional practice to maintain labor analgesia with a combination of continuous epidural infusion and patient-controlled epidural analgesia using an automated epidural pump, compelling data now shows that bolus injection through the epidural catheter may result in better distribution of anesthetic solution in the epidural space. The programmed intermittent epidural bolus technique is proposed as a better maintenance mode and may represent a more effective mode of maintaining epidural analgesia for labor, especially prolonged labor. Additional prospective and adequately powered studies are needed to confirm findings and determine the optimal combination of volume, rate, time, and drug concentration.

> Obstetric hemorrhage remains the leading cause of maternal death and severe morbidity worldwide. Although uterine atony is the most common cause of peripartum bleeding, abnormal placentation, coagulation disorders, and genital tract trauma contribute to adverse maternal outcomes. Given the inability to reliably predict patients at high risk for obstetric hemorrhage, all parturients should be considered susceptible, and extreme vigilance must be exercised in the assessment of blood loss and hemodynamic stability during the peripartum period. Obstetric-specific hemorrhage protocols, facilitating the integration and timely escalation of pharmacologic, radiological, surgical, and transfusion interventions, are critical to the successful management of peripartum bleeding.

> This article provides an overview of the use of ultrasonography in obstetric anesthesia. It discusses the indications, benefits, and techniques of using ultrasonography to optimize the delivery of anesthesia and provide safe and efficacious clinical care. More specifically, it discusses the use of ultrasonography to facilitate neuraxial anesthesia, abdominal field blocks, central and

peripheral vascular access, as well as the assessment of the lung fields and gastric contents, and identification of the cricothyroid membrane.

Emily McQuaid-Hanson and May C.M. Pian-Smith

Interprofessional teams work together on the labor and delivery unit, where clinical care is often unscheduled, rapidly evolving, and fast paced. Effective communication is key for coordinated delivery of optimal care and for fostering a culture of community and safety in the workplace. The preoperative huddle allows for information sharing, cross-checking, and preparation before the start of surgery. Postoperative debriefings allow the operative team to engage in ongoing process improvement. Debriefings after adverse events allow for shared understanding, mutual healing, and help mitigating the harm to potential "second victims."

Annemaria De Tina and Arvind Palanisamy

Rodent studies on the effect of general anesthesia during the third trimester on neurocognitive outcomes are mixed, but primate studies suggest that a clinically relevant exposure to anesthetic agents during the third trimester can trigger neuronal and glial cell death. Human studies are conflicting and the evidence is weak. This is an up-to-date review of the literature on the neurodevelopmental effects of anesthetic agents administered during the third trimester. Early brain development and critical periods of neurodevelopment as it relates to neurotoxicity are highlighted. Rodent, nonhuman primate, and population studies are discussed and placed in the context of clinical practice.

Stephanie Lim and Jennifer Lucero

Breech presentation is the most common abnormal fetal presentation and complicates approximately 3% to 4% of all pregnancies. External cephalic version (ECV) should be recommended to women with a breech singleton pregnancy, if there is no maternal or fetal contraindication. ECV increases the chance of cephalic presentation at the onset of labor and decreases the rate of cesarean delivery by almost 40%. The success rate of ECV is approximately 60%. Review of the risks and benefits for performing an ECV and for both the timing of ECV and the number of attempts should be should be discussed with the patient.

Nerlyne K. Dhariwal and Grant C. Lynde

Hypertensive disorders of pregnancy complicate approximately 10% of all deliveries in the United States and are a leading cause of maternal and fetal morbidity and mortality. Preeclampsia is defined as hypertension in association with proteinuria, thrombocytopenia, impaired liver function, renal insufficiency, pulmonary edema, or new-onset cerebral or visual disturbances. The greatest risk factor for the development of preeclampsia is a history of preeclampsia. There currently is no effective means for the prevention of preeclampsia. Approximately 39% of patients diagnosed with preeclampsia have hypertension and approximately 20% have proteinuria 3 months postpartum. Preeclampsia increases the risk of patients developing hypertension later in life.

Cesarean delivery rates are increasing worldwide, and effective postoperative pain management is a key priority of women undergoing cesarean delivery. Inadequate pain management in the acute postoperative period is associated with persistent pain, greater opioid use, delayed functional recovery, and increased postpartum depression. In addition to pain relief, optimal management of patients after cesarean delivery should address the goals of unrestricted maternal mobility, minimal maternal and neonatal side effects, rapid recovery to baseline functionality, and early discharge home. Multimodal analgesia should include neuraxial morphine in conjunction with nonopioid adjuncts, with additional oral or intravenous opioids reserved for severe breakthrough pain.

Nitrous oxide, long used during labor in Europe, is gaining popularity in the United States. It offers many beneficial attributes, with few drawbacks. Cost, safety, and side effect profiles are favorable. Analgesic effectiveness is highly variable, yet maternal satisfaction is often high among the women who choose to use it. Despite being less effective in treating labor pain than neuraxial analgesic modalities, nitrous oxide serves the needs and preferences of a subset of laboring parturients. Nitrous oxide should, therefore, be considered for inclusion in the repertoire of modalities used to alleviate pain and facilitate effective coping during labor.

Awareness during general anesthesia for cesarean delivery continues to be a major problem. The key to preventing awareness is strict attention to anesthetic technique. The prevalence and implications of aortocaval compression have been firmly established. Compression of the vena cava is a real occurrence when assuming the supine position. Relief of this compression most likely does not occur until the patient is turned 30°, which is not feasible for performing cesarean delivery. Although it is still wise to tilt the patient, the benefit of this tilt may not be as great as once thought.

Headache after dural puncture is a common complication accompanying neuraxial anesthesia. The proposed cause is loss of cerebrospinal fluid through the puncture into the epidural space. Although obstetric patients are at risk for the development of this headache because of female gender and young age, there is a difference in the obstetric population. Women who deliver by cesarean delivery have a lower incidence of headache after dural puncture compared with those who deliver vaginally. Treatment of postdural puncture headache is an epidural blood patch. Departments should develop protocols for management of accidental dural puncture, including appropriate follow-up and indications for further management.

ANESTHESIOLOGY CLINICS

RELATED INTEREST

Critical Care Clinics, January 2016 (Vol. 32, No. 1)
Obstetric and Gynecologic Emergencies
Susan E. Dantoni and Peter J. Papadakos, *Editors*
Available at: http://www.criticalcare.theclinics.com/

THE CLINICS ARE AVAILABLE ONLINE!
Access your subscription at:
www.theclinics.com

Foreword

Anesthesiologists in Obstetric Care: Beyond Labor Epidurals and C-Section Care

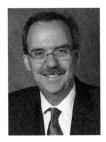

Lee A. Fleisher, MD, FACC
Consulting Editor

Anesthesiology is moving toward perioperative medicine. In the Obstetric arena, this could simply focus on the time around delivery, but there are opportunities for anesthesiologists to focus on the period before delivery and beyond this acute 24- to 72-hour time period. In thinking about our ability to enhance obstetric care, the current editors have expanded the articles to include these time periods. They have also included an article on the implications of anesthesia on the developing fetus. The current series of articles helps define best practices and our ability to influence care and serve our obstetric patients.

This issue was proposed by a leader in thought in this arena and previous editor on this topic, Robert R. Gaiser, MD, MSEd. Dr Gaiser is Professor and Chair of Anesthesiology at the University of Kentucky. He is the past President of the Society for Obstetric Anesthesia and Perinatology and a leader in Obstetric anesthesiology. He is also an expert in education and is Chair of the Anesthesiology Residency Review Committee and a member of the American Board of Anesthesiology. He has enlisted a former colleague from the University of Pennsylvania, Onyi Onuoha, MD, MPH, to assist in editing this issue. Dr Onuoha completed a fellowship in obstetric anesthesia and focused on both quality improvement and education in obstetric anesthetic care. Together,

Anesthesiology Clin 35 (2017) xiii–xiv
http://dx.doi.org/10.1016/j.anclin.2016.12.002
1932-2275/17/© 2016 Published by Elsevier Inc.

they have brought together a phenomenal group of authors to educate us on best current practices.

Lee A. Fleisher, MD, FACC
Perelman School of Medicine
University of Pennsylvania
3400 Spruce Street, Dulles 680
Philadelphia, PA 19104, USA

E-mail address:
Lee.Fleisher@uphs.upenn.edu

Preface

Embracing the Next Phase in Obstetric Anesthesiology

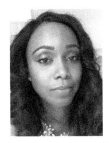
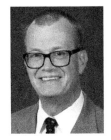

Onyi C. Onuoha, MD, MPH   Robert R. Gaiser, MD
Editors

The accreditation of obstetric anesthesia by the Accreditation Council for Graduate Medical Education in the United States is the next phase in the evolution of the specialty. Prior to accreditation, the amount of scholarship, education, and research discovery in the field had been substantial with the practice addressing pertinent questions relating to the anesthetic implications in high-risk pregnancy; complications of pregnancy-related diseases; preterm labor; advances in labor analgesia; the use of noninvasive technology in labor and delivery; postcesarean analgesia; patient safety; fetal development; and advances in neonatology. With the ability to introduce structure and create national standards for fellows through the accreditation of the specialty, the next phase presents more opportunities for growth and innovation in research in the field of obstetric anesthesia.

Pioneering these efforts to educate the next generation are dedicated clinicians and researchers who continue to address challenging and pertinent questions by performing novel evidence-based research ranging from the primary care of the parturient to the use of noninvasive cutting-edge technology to improve the care of the parturient. With the changing demographics of the obstetric population, "the critically ill parturient," the field of obstetric anesthesia is continually evolving. The advancement of the specialty reflects the changing role of the obstetric anesthesiologist from a primarily procedural expert to a well-versed perioperative clinician collaborating with the nurse, obstetrician, neonatologist, and other consulting specialists in the multidisciplinary setting.

We are therefore thrilled to have such a talented group of experts contributing to this issue of *Anesthesiology Clinics* by addressing some of the relevant questions in obstetric anesthesia. This issue represents a comprehensive review, description, and update of current topics that add new knowledge to the field of obstetric anesthesia with the primary goal of improving maternal and fetal outcomes during pregnancy and the postpartum period. Additional insight is provided on controversial and debated topics like

Anesthesiology Clin 35 (2017) xv–xvi
http://dx.doi.org/10.1016/j.anclin.2016.12.001
1932-2275/17/© 2016 Published by Elsevier Inc.

the link between neurocognitive outcomes and general anesthesia during the third trimester; the comparison between continuous epidural infusion and programmed intermittent epidural bolus for labor analgesia; the use of nitrous oxide in the laboring patient; obstetric versus anesthesia approaches to external cephalic version; and the current evidence on tilts and full stomach in patients undergoing cesarean delivery. Updates are included on ever-changing subject areas, such as the management of patients with preeclampsia, prophylaxis and management of obstetric hemorrhage, and the optimal pain management after cesarean delivery. And finally, topics delineating the future direction of obstetric anesthesia as in the use of ultrasound in obstetric anesthesia and huddles/debriefing to improve communication on labor and delivery are integrated in the content list. Ultimately, this issue highlights the various roles of the obstetric anesthesiologist in the care of the parturient.

We are grateful to all our contributors for their willingness to dedicate their time and effort writing this issue despite their busy schedules. We especially want to dedicate this issue to Dr Lee A. Fleisher, Chair of Anesthesia at the Hospital of the University of Pennsylvania and consulting editor, for his continuous support, mentorship, and investment in promoting education and research for resident and faculty development. Although not an obstetric anesthesiologist, his dedication to the growth of the specialty and scholarly pursuit as a whole inspires us and increases our drive to be more visibly well-rounded perioperative clinicians for the benefit and safety of our patients.

Onyi C. Onuoha, MD, MPH
Department of Anesthesiology
and Critical Care
Perelman School of Medicine
University of Pennsylvania
3400 Spruce Street, Dulles 6
Philadelphia, PA 19104, USA

Robert R. Gaiser, MD
Department of Anesthesiology
University of Kentucky
Lexington, KY 40506, USA

E-mail addresses:
Onyi.Onuoha@uphs.upenn.edu (O.C. Onuoha)
robert.gaiser@uky.edu (R.R. Gaiser)

Epidural Analgesia for Labor

Continuous Infusion Versus Programmed Intermittent Bolus

Onyi C. Onuoha, MD, MPH

KEYWORDS

- Neuraxial analgesia • Labor • Epidural • Combined-spinal epidural (CSE)
- Automated pump • Continuous epidural infusion (CEI)
- Programmed intermittent epidural bolus (PIEB)
- Patient-controlled epidural analgesia (PCEA)

KEY POINTS

- The programmed intermittent epidural bolus (PIEB) technique, as a maintenance mode for labor analgesia, may offer multiple benefits over the current traditional continuous infusion technique.
- Proposed benefits of the PIEB technique, as indicated by multiple studies, include the use of less local anesthetic and opioids, the occurrence of less breakthrough pain, improved patient satisfaction, and a lower incidence of both motor block and instrumental vaginal delivery.
- Fine-tuning appropriate algorithms using advanced pump technology in tandem with studies to determine the optimal combination of volume, rate, time interval, and drug concentrations are needed to improve the use of the intermittent bolus technique in clinical practice.
- More studies are necessary to consistently demonstrate an improvement in labor analgesia, and maternal and fetal obstetric outcomes with the intermittent bolus technique.

INTRODUCTION: LABOR ANALGESIA

Although once controversial, the current preferred use of neuraxial analgesic techniques by anesthesiologists, obstetricians and patients for labor, has almost established these modalities as the standard of care for labor pain in developed countries such as the United States. The use of neuraxial techniques, such as epidural and combined spinal-epidural (CSE) analgesia, has been shown to be the most effective

Department of Anesthesiology and Critical Care, Perelman School of Medicine, Hospital of the University of Pennsylvania, 3400 Spruce Street, Dulles 6, Philadelphia, PA 19104, USA
E-mail address: Onyi.Onuoha@uphs.upenn.edu

Anesthesiology Clin 35 (2017) 1–14
http://dx.doi.org/10.1016/j.anclin.2016.09.003
1932-2275/17/© 2016 Elsevier Inc. All rights reserved.
anesthesiology.theclinics.com

modality for pain relief in labor.[1] In addition to providing analgesic benefits to the mother, neuraxial analgesia can be converted to surgical anesthesia if operative delivery is required.[2,3]

The updated guidelines for labor analgesia, as proposed by the American Society of Anesthesiologists (ASA) Task Force and Committee on Standards and Practice Parameters in 2016, recommend that the choice of analgesic technique depend on the medical status of the patient, anesthetic risk factors, obstetric risk factors, patient preferences, progress of labor, and resources at the facility. With sufficient resources, neuraxial analgesic techniques should be offered among the analgesic options for labor with the primary goal of providing adequate maternal analgesia with minimal motor block (eg, achieved with the administration of local anesthetics at low concentrations with or without opioids).[4] Guidelines advocate the use of dilute concentrations of local anesthetics with opioids to produce as little motor block as possible. A local anesthetic may be added to a spinal opioid to increase duration and improve the quality of analgesia. A catheter technique should be considered if labor is expected to last longer than the analgesic effects of the spinal drugs chosen, or if there is a good possibility of operative delivery.[4] CSE techniques may be used to provide effective and rapid onset of analgesia for labor. Patient controlled epidural analgesia (PCEA) may be used to provide an effective and flexible approach for the maintenance of labor analgesia. The use of PCEA may be preferable to fixed-rate continuous infusion epidural for providing fewer anesthetic interventions and reducing dosages of local anesthetics. PCEA may be used with or without a background infusion.[4]

In many institutions in North America and Europe, neuraxial labor analgesia is initiated with a local anesthetic and an opioid using the epidural or CSE technique. Maintenance regimens have evolved from manual boluses by the clinician to continuous infusions alone and, subsequently, with patient-controlled boluses through a pump.[5] PCEA with or without a background continuous epidural infusion (CEI) is currently the most used technique.[5] The current maintenance regimen consists of a combination of a local anesthetic with an opioid administered through an epidural catheter using an automated epidural pump. Given that most providers support the use of neuraxial analgesia for labor, it is crucial that attempts are made to optimize the different techniques available for the maintenance of analgesia throughout labor.

The benefits of the CEI and programmed intermittent epidural bolus (PIEB) techniques for labor analgesia are reviewed in this article. In addition, the clinical implications and challenges encountered with each technique, and current controversies and areas for further research will be discussed to maximize the effective use of these analgesic modalities for labor pain.

MAINTENANCE OF LABOR ANALGESIA

Once labor analgesia is established by using an epidural or CSE technique, maintenance of analgesia can be achieved with[1] (1) CEI or (2) PIEB, each supplemented by the use of (3) PCEA (**Table 1**).

Continuous Epidural Infusion

In the past, CEI compared with manual intermittent boluses by the anesthesiologist or with PCEA alone, had been associated with a more consistent and smoother analgesia, improved patient satisfaction, and reduced workload for the anesthesiologist.[6] The traditional practice, therefore, has involved maintaining epidural analgesia for labor with the combination of a local anesthetic and opioid administered via CEI with the use of PCEA for breakthrough pain.[7] However, the utility of CEI for maintenance of

Table 1
Outcomes and clinical implications

Technique	Advantages	Clinical Implications
PIEB + PCEA	1. ↓Total drug (local anesthetic) used 2. ↓Total drug (opioid) used 3. ↓Incidence of motor block 4. ↓Incidence of instrumental vaginal delivery 5. ↓Breakthrough pain (fewer request for additional PCEA/clinician boluses) 6. ↑Patient satisfaction	↓Incidence of motor block ↓Systemic absorption, hence ↓risk of fetal respiratory depression ↓Incidence of forceps and vacuum-assisted vaginal delivery, ↑maternal satisfaction ↓Adverse effects of instrumental delivery (sphincter tears, fecal incontinence, fetal injury, postpartum pain) ↑Maternal satisfaction ↓Clinician workload on a busy labor and delivery unit May return to medical practice for subsequent deliveries, may recommend institution to friends
	Disadvantages (of manual boluses or PCEA alone) 1. Frequent provider interventions required 2. Waxing and waning intervals of analgesia and pain relief 3. Safety implications with high bolus doses	[a]Evident with nonoptimal PIEB settings or manual boluses → ↓Maternal satisfaction, ↑physician workload Safer administering potentially toxic drugs as an infusion rather than a bolus → ↑risk of adverse drug reaction (eg, local anesthetic toxicity, high or total spinal)
CEI + PCEA	*Advantages (compared with manual boluses or PCEA alone)* 1. More consistent analgesia, smoother analgesic experience for the parturient 2. Fewer medical interventions 3. ↓Workload for the anesthesiologist *Disadvantages* 1. Regression of sensory block overtime 2. Need for regular rescue medication 3. ↑Incidence of motor block due to larger local anesthetic volumes (↑hourly consumption) 4. ↑Incidence of instrumental vaginal delivery	[a]CEI compared with manual intermittent boluses or PCEA alone before the advent of the programmed intermittent bolus technique ↑Need for higher infusion rates or regular top-ups ↓Patient satisfaction, ↑physician workload ↓Pelvic muscle tone, difficulty with internal rotation of fetal head ↑Adverse effects of instrumental delivery (sphincter tears, fecal incontinence, fetal injury, postpartum pain)

Based on most of the studies.
↑ (increase in), ↓ (decrease in), → (resulting in).
[a] Comparisons made to manual intermittent boluses or PCEA alone before the advent of the PIEB technique.

labor analgesia has been challenged by several studies within the last decade due to its association with greater local anesthetic consumption and the frequent need for rescue boluses.[7,8] Higher infusion rates to decrease the need for rescue boluses subsequently result in an increase in the degree of maternal motor block possibly contributing to increased rates of instrumental deliveries and shoulder dystocia.[7,8] Constant infusion of epidural solution may also result in progressive regression of the block, with resultant failure of pain control, and an increase in physician workload.[9] Although an alternative mode of delivery, the PIEB technique, had been proposed by several studies, CEI remained the traditional practice in most facilities due to the initial lack of the automated pump technology capable of delivering preset intermittent epidural boluses (IEBs) along with the PCEA.

Programmed Intermittent Epidural Bolus

The PIEB technique is an automated method of administering epidural solutions at fixed boluses and scheduled intervals. It can be used as an alternative to CEI alone or as a background administration with the PCEA technique.[5] Several studies comparing the PIEB plus (+) PCEA technique with the CEI + PCEA technique have concluded that the automated bolus technique is generally superior to the continuous technique providing either equal or better analgesia with less drug.[10] Decreased motor block and, consequently, a decreased need for instrumental delivery have also been associated with this maintenance technique.[1]

The exact mechanism responsible for this difference is, however, not fully understood.[10] Possible explanations have been proposed to support the advantages of intermittent bolus compared with continuous infusion administration of epidural solutions. Cadaveric dissections with cryomicrotome sectioning have shown a more uniform spread of liquid in the epidural space, through the intervertebral foramina, and along the nerve sheaths when using large volumes of injectate at high injection pressures.[11] This suggests that epidural solutions spread more evenly when injected as a bolus than as a continuous infusion.[11] Additionally, epidural bolus through a multiorifice catheter may result in a wider sensory blockade compared with a continuous infusion of the same volume in which the infusion primarily exits through the proximal orifice.[12] Current clinical data, however, show some mixed results, and do not support or refute greater spread of anesthetic solution by intermittent bolus as the principal mechanism of reduced analgesia consumption.[10] Furthermore, Capogna and colleagues,[1] and Capogna and Stirparo,[8] attempted to describe differences in the dynamics of nerve block with intermittent or continuous infusion administration that may contribute to the findings previously cited. Analgesia and motor block are produced by the movement of local anesthetic from the extraneural space into the nerve along a diffusion gradient. Over time, equilibrium or a steady state is achieved; however, nerve blockade is overcome when the intraneural concentration exceeds the extraneural concentration and the diffusion gradient is reversed. With low concentrations of local anesthetic given in intermittent boluses, blockade of motor fibers (thick, long-internode fibers) is unlikely given the insufficient total amount of local anesthetic inside the nerve. With continuous infusion, however, not only is the extraneural concentration of local anesthetic generally persistently higher than in the intraneural space, the total concentration inside the nerve is increased, thus reaching the threshold for motor fiber block.[1,8]

The technology for PIEB is relatively new and has been minimally studied over the last decade.[7] With the recent development of upgraded software to support the automated administration of epidural maintenance solutions via PIEB, special pumps[7] can now be used in routine practice for administering maintenance solutions using the bolus technique. Until recently, the continuous technique alone had been used due to the lack of automated pumps facilitating the delivery of the combined regimen (timed boluses with PCEA). In addition, most randomized studies advocating for the PIEB technique used the 2-pump system per parturient during the investigative process, which may not equate exactly to a 1-pump system with the ability to deliver both modes. The availability of such pumps provides researchers with the opportunity to make comparisons of maintenance techniques with the actual pump technology used in clinical practice.

The new pump is able to deliver boluses at a higher flow rate and has different interactions between the PIEB interval and the PCEA lockout interval. Hence, outcomes using these new practical pumps may be different from previous studies.[7] With the old software, the maximum infusion rate was 175 mL per hour. The new software allows for rates of up to 250 mL per hour with the standard tubing and 500 mL per hour with the special high-flow tubing.[7] In addition, with the 2-pump system, the lockout period of the PIEB was independent of that of the PCEA. Using 1 pump for drug administration ensures the option to choose either the PCEA or the PIEB lockout periods as the interval between a PIEB and a PCEA dose. Automated systems designed to administer a bolus at programmable intervals are believed to combine the advantages of both manual bolus and combined infusion.[1]

Supplementary: Patient-Controlled Epidural Analgesia

The PCEA is a top-up technique in which the patient administers a bolus of epidural solution at irregular intervals as analgesia wanes and pain returns.[8] It has been shown to decrease breakthrough pain requiring physician top-ups, reduce local anesthetic consumption without compromising analgesic efficacy, and increase patient autonomy and satisfaction during labor.[13] Cultural factors, maternal training, and expectations affect the efficacy of this technique.[8] The goal of the anesthesiologist in the maintenance of labor analgesia is to prevent pain reoccurrence by administering the anesthetic solution before the pain returns. Hence, maintenance techniques that deliver anesthetic solutions continuously (CEI) or at regular intervals (PIEB) are often used in addition to the PCEA top-up technique, with the latter mostly aimed at targeting breakthrough pain. Recent studies investigating the optimal technique for maintaining epidural labor analgesia have incorporated the use of PCEA for supplementary analgesia. The PCEA was mostly used in addition to PIEB and CEI (via 2 separate pumps in recent studies)[1,5,7,10,12,13] for breakthrough pain relief. Halpern and Carvalho[14] (2009) compared 7 randomized clinical trials on PCEA with and without background infusions. Although lower consumption of local anesthetic was reported in women who received PCEA alone, none of the other outcomes (maternal analgesia, maternal satisfaction, clinician workload, unscheduled clinician interventions, motor block) were significantly better in subjects who received PCEA without the basal infusion. Even though Sezer and Gunaydin[15] (2007) demonstrated that the demand-only PCEA regimen alone provided satisfactory maintenance analgesia, there has been no consensus on the use of this mode as an adequate and optimal maintenance analgesic regimen for labor.

CURRENT EVIDENCE AND LITERATURE REVIEW: SOME SEMINAL STUDIES

Several studies within the last decade have attempted to explore the efficacy of both maintenance techniques for labor analgesia. These studies have ranged from randomized controlled trials to meta-analyses and retrospective reviews of electronic medical record. Some seminal recent studies are reviewed in the following sections.

Wong and Colleagues (2006)

Wong and colleagues[12] (2006) compared data from 126 healthy term women with singleton pregnancies (63 per group) in which labor analgesia was initiated using the CSE technique (bupivacaine 1.25 mg and fentanyl 15 µg + epidural test dose: lidocaine 45 mg + epinephrine 15 µg) and thereafter maintained with either (1) PIEB (6 mL bolus every 30 minutes starting at 45 minutes after intrathecal dose) + PCEA or (2) CEI (12 mL per hour starting at 15 minutes after the intrathecal dose) + PCEA using a 2-pump system. The primary outcome variable was bupivacaine consumption per hour of infusion. Results showed that the median total bupivacaine delivered per hour of infusion was less in the PIEB group (10.5 mg/h) compared with the CEI group (12.3 mg/h, $P<.01$) even after controlling for the basal dose of bupivacaine per hour administered by the PIEB pump compared with the CEI pump. The median fentanyl dose per hour of infusion was also less in the PIEB group compared with the CEI group. The number of subjects requiring manual rescue boluses, the number of manual rescue boluses per subject, and the amount of bupivacaine given with the manual rescue boluses were less in the PIEB group. Interestingly, despite decreased bupivacaine consumption, labor pain as measured via hourly visual analog pain scale (VAPS), time to first PCEA request, number of requests, and delivered PCEA boluses of bupivacaine were similar between groups. Subject satisfaction with pain management was greater in the PIEB group compared with the CEI group.

Summary

The investigators concluded that PIEB + PCEA resulted in less bupivacaine consumption and higher subject satisfaction compared with CEI + PCEA, while providing equivalent labor analgesia. This difference, however, was greater in subjects with labor of longer duration.

Fettes and Colleagues (2006)

Fettes and colleagues[9] (2006) compared 40 ASA I-II primigravid full-term subjects in a randomized, double-blind trial in which labor analgesia was initiated by an epidural loading bolus of plain ropivacaine 0.2% 15 to 20 mL titrated until analgesia and bilateral sensory block T10. Thereafter, subjects were randomized to receive ropivacaine 2 mg/mL with fentanyl 2 µg/mL either as

1. continuous infusion (control group, started immediately at a rate of 10 mL/h) or
2. intermittent administration (study group, started 30 minutes after time zero, hourly boluses of 10 mL delivered at 2 mL/min).

The study was primarily designed to measure the efficacy of analgesia during the first stage of labor. Subjects in the continuous group required more than 3 times more epidural boluses to maintain pain relief compared with the intermittent group ($P = .02$). The mean dose of ropivacaine adjusted for time was significantly less for the intermittent group than the continuous group (64.3 mg vs 72.7 mg, $P<.01$). Duration of uninterrupted analgesia (time to first rescue bolus) was longer in the intermittent group ($P<.02$). Sensory spread and motor block were similar in the 2 groups.

Summary

The investigators concluded that the intermittent technique was more efficacious due to fewer supplementary injections and less total drug to maintain similar pain scores. The investigators, however, failed to show any difference in pain scores (primary outcome measure) or sensory or motor block between the 2 groups.

Leo and Colleagues (2010)

Leo and colleagues[13] (2010) recruited 62 healthy term nulliparous women with singleton pregnancies and labor analgesia was initiated using the CSE technique (ropivacaine

2 mg and fentanyl 15 µg + epidural catheter flushed with 3 mL of 1.5% lidocaine). Subjects were thereafter randomized to receive 0.1% ropivacaine with 2 µg/mL of fentanyl either by (1). PCEA with a continuous basal infusion BI (Group PCEA + BI = 5 mL/h started immediately after intrathecal drug administration) or (2). PCEA with automated mandatory boluses AMB (Group PCEA + AMB = 5 mL/hr starting at 30 minutes after the intrathecal dose). The primary outcome of interest was the incidence of breakthrough pain requiring physician top-up. Secondary variables included time-weighted local anesthetic consumption, maternal satisfaction scores, and duration of effective analgesia post-CSE. There was no difference in the incidence of breakthrough pain requiring physician epidural top-up in both groups. Although the numbers were too small for meaningful statistical analysis, the median cervical dilation at which breakthrough pain occurred was greater in group PCEA + AMB compared with group PCEA + BI. The time-weighted hourly consumption of ropivacaine, including maintenance doses, subject-administered and clinician-administered boluses, was significantly lower in the PCEA + AMB group (mean, 7.6 mL, SD = 3.2) compared with the PCEA + BI group (mean 9.3 mL, SD = 2.5, $P<.001$). The mean time to first PCEA self-bolus post-CSE was significantly longer in the PCEA + AMB group (268 minutes) compared with the PCEA + BI (104 minutes) group ($P<.001$). Parturients in both groups had similar mean durations of labor. Subjects in group PCEA + AMB rated their overall labor analgesia experience better (satisfaction) than those in group PCEA + BI ($P<.001$).

Summary

The investigators concluded that the PCEA with automated mandatory boluses provided greater maternal satisfaction and longer duration of effective analgesia than the PCEA with infusion despite reduced analgesic consumption. The investigators, however, failed to show any difference in the incidence of breakthrough pain requiring physician top-up (primary outcome measure) between the 2 groups.

Capogna and Colleagues (2011)

Capogna and colleagues[1] (2011) compared 145 healthy, nulliparous, term women in a randomized, double-blind, controlled study in which labor analgesia was initiated by an epidural loading bolus consisting of 20 mL 0.0625% levobupivacaine (L-bupiv) + 10 µg sufentanil and, thereafter, subjects were randomized to receive a maintenance dose of either (1) PIEB (10 mL of 0.0625% L-bupiv + 0.5 µg/mL of sufentanil every hour beginning 60 minutes after loading dose) + PCEA or (2) CEI (rate of 10 mL/h beginning immediately after loading dose) + PCEA using the 2-pump system per parturient. The PCEA was programmed to deliver 5 mL subject-activated boluses of L-bupiv 0.125% with a lockout interval of 10 minutes and a per hour maximum volume of 15 mL. The primary endpoint was the incidence of motor block with a secondary endpoint of the incidence of instrumental vaginal delivery. PIEB resulted in less motor block (2.7%) in the parturient during labor and at full cervical dilation compared with the CEI group (37%, $P<.001$). In addition, motor block occurred earlier in subjects who received CEI than those receiving PIEB. The occurrence of motor block at full cervical dilation was associated with an increased risk of instrumental delivery (vacuum-assisted, $P = .002$, odds ratio [OR] 230, CI 8–889). However, there was no difference in the cesarean delivery rate between the groups. The total L-bupiv + sufentanil consumption, number of subjects requiring additional PCEA boluses, and mean number of PCEA boluses per subject were lower in the PIEB group ($P<.001$). Labor pain, as assessed by hourly VAPS scores was similar between both groups.

Summary

The investigators concluded that the maintenance of labor analgesia with PIEB resulted in a lower incidence of maternal motor block (primary endpoint) and instrumental vaginal delivery compared with CEI.

Wong and Colleagues (2011)

Wong and colleagues[10] (2011) aimed to quantify the optimal combination of bolus volume and dosing interval by comparing 190 healthy, term, nulliparous women in a randomized, double-blind study in which labor analgesia was initiated with a CSE consisting of 1.25 mg of intrathecal bupivacaine with 15 μg of fentanyl and test dose administered through the epidural catheter (lidocaine 45 mg + epinephrine 15 μg). Subjects were thereafter randomized into 1 of 3 PIEB groups with an epidural maintenance regimen of 0.625 mg/mL bupivacaine with fentanyl 1.95 μg/mL and the first bolus initiated 30 minutes after the intrathecal bolus dose. Groups included (1) PIEB equals (=) 2.5 mL every 15 minutes (2.5/15), (2) PIEB = 5 mL every 30 minutes (5/30), and (3) PIEB = 10 mL every 60 minutes (10/60). A second PCEA pump was set at a bolus dose of 5 mL at 150 mL per hour, lockout interval at 10 minutes, no basal infusion rate, and a maximum dose of 15 mL per hour for all groups. The primary outcome was total bupivacaine consumption per hour of labor analgesia. Results showed that subjects randomized to group 10/60 consumed less total bupivacaine (median, 8.8 mg) compared with women in groups 2.5/15 (10.4 mg) and 5/30 (10.0 mg), $P = .005$. The amount of fentanyl per hour of labor consumed was not different among groups. There were no differences among groups in PCEA requests or administrations, number of manual bolus doses for breakthrough pain, time to first PCEA dose or manual dose, or subject satisfaction with labor analgesia. There was also no difference in either the cephalad extent of sensory analgesia to ice or pressure sensory threshold to von Frey filament at several dermatomes.

Summary

The investigators concluded that extending the PIEB interval and volume from 15 to 60 minutes, and 2.5 mL to 10 mL, respectively decreased bupivacaine consumption without decreasing subject satisfaction. They also indicated that although the larger volume administration at a longer interval resulted in less bupivacaine than smaller volumes at shorter intervals, the difference in bupivacaine consumption is unlikely to be clinically relevant when using low concentration solutions that result in minimal or no motor blockade.

George and Colleagues (2013)

George and colleagues[16] (2013) performed a systematic review of 9 randomized controlled trials involving 694 subjects in whom the effect of IEB was compared with the current standard CEI dosing with or without PCEA. Based on the hypothesis that CEI may involve large doses of local anesthetic resulting in profound motor blockade and subsequent instrumental deliveries, the primary outcome measures evaluated included subject satisfaction, the need for manual anesthesia interventions, labor progression, and the mode of delivery in healthy women receiving labor epidural analgesia. Secondary outcomes were degree of motor blockade, degree of sensory blockade, time to first anesthetic intervention, local anesthetic dose delivered per hour, presence of maternal adverse effects, neonatal Apgar scores at 1 minute and 5 minutes, and umbilical artery and vein pH. Both techniques of local anesthesia delivery were comparable in terms of total duration of labor but there was a statistically significant reduction in the length of the second stage of labor (as much as 22 minutes shorter) with IEB. The use of IEB resulted in a small but statistically significant reduction in local anesthetic usage (mean difference [MD], −1.2 mg bupivacaine equivalent per hour; 95% CI, −2.2 to −0.3). There was however no statistical difference between IEB and CEI in the rate of cesarean delivery (OR, 0.87; 95% CI, 0.56–1.35), duration of labor (MD, −17 minutes; 95% CI, −42 to 7), or the need for anesthetic intervention (OR, 0.56; 95% CI, 0.29–1.06). Maternal satisfaction score (100 mm VAPS) was higher with IEB (MD 7.0 mm, 95% CI 6.2–7.8).

Summary
The investigators concluded that the current evidence suggests a slight reduction of local anesthetic usage and improvement in maternal satisfaction by IEB. The pooled data for instrumental delivery rate, rate of anesthetic interventions, and duration of labor each had wide a confidence interval that contained clinically significant end points, therefore prohibiting definitive conclusions. There remains a potential that IEB improves instrumental delivery rate and the need of anesthesia interventions.

McKenzie and Colleagues (2016)

McKenzie and colleagues[5] (2016) conducted a retrospective review of the electronic medical records for vaginal deliveries with neuraxial analgesia before and after the introduction of PIEB at an academic university medical institution. Labor analgesia was initiated with either 15 mL of epidural 0.125% bupivacaine + sufentanil 10 µg or CSE with intrathecal bupivacaine 2.5 mg + sufentanil 5 µg. Maintenance technique for labor analgesia transitioned from CEI (0.0625% bupivacaine + sufentanil 0.4 µg/mL at 12 mL/h + PCEA 0/12/15) to PIEB (9 mL every 45 minutes starting 30 minutes after pump initiation + PCEA 0/10/10) in October 2014. The primary outcome was the proportion of women requiring a clinician rescue bolus during labor. Secondary outcomes included mean and highest verbal pain score during labor, number of clinician boluses needed, total clinician bolus dose, incidence of unilateral pain or sensory level, hypotension requiring anesthetic intervention, and mode of delivery. Results showed a significant difference in the primary outcome measure with fewer women in the PIEB group requiring a clinician rescue bolus during labor (12% vs 19%, $P = .012$). Time to first clinician bolus after epidural placement, number of clinician boluses received and the total dose given among the subjects who required clinician boluses did not differ between the groups. Unilateral block was 5.4% in the CEI group and 1.8% in the PIEB group ($P = .021$). The mode of delivery did not differ between groups.

Summary
The investigators concluded that PIEB used in conjunction with PCEA reduced the number of women requiring clinician rescue boluses (primary outcome measure) while providing comparable labor analgesia as CEI.

Tien and Colleagues (2016)

Tien and colleagues[7] (2016) performed a retrospective comparison of 528 subjects from an academic university medical center who received maintenance of epidural labor analgesia via PIEB or CEI using the CADD-Solis v3.0 pump (single pump) to assess whether the use of PIEB is associated with decreased local anesthetic consumption, decreased PCEA use, and decreased rescue analgesia requirements compared with CEI. The neuraxial regimen used to initiate labor analgesia consisted of bupivacaine 0.125 mg/mL with fentanyl 2 μg/mL. All subjects identified were categorized into 3 groups:

1. CEI 5 mL per hour
2. PIEB 5 mL per 60 minutes
3. PIEB 3 mL per 30 minutes.

All subjects had similar PCEA settings. The PIEB delivery rate was set at 250 mL per hour and the lockout interval between the PIEB and PCEA doses was set at the PCEA lockout interval of 8 minutes. The primary endpoint was total volume of local anesthetics consumed per hour. Secondary outcome measures were need for clinician boluses, pattern of PCEA use, degree of motor blockade, and delivery mode. Overall, there was no significant difference in patterns of local anesthetic use among the 3 groups. Results showed the median local anesthetic consumed was 10.3, 9.5, and 9.7 mL per hour, respectively ($P = .10$). There were also no differences in the number of rescue clinician boluses or PCEA attempts per hour but total PCEA volume per hour and ratio of PCEA attempted or given were significantly different among the groups with the PIEB 3 mL per 30 minutes using lower PCEA volume than the CEI group ($P = .04$). Groups PIEB 3 mL per 30 minutes and PIEB 5 mL per 60 minutes had higher ratio of PCEA attempts to PCEA boluses given per hour than the CEI group ($P<.01$ and $P = .01$, respectively). There were no differences in Bromage scores ($P = .14$) or delivery mode ($P = .55$) among the groups.

Summary
The investigators concluded through this retrospective study (limitations: single-center, retrospective design, no randomization) that the epidural maintenance regimen used (CEI vs PIEB) was not associated with differences in local anesthetic consumption, delivery mode, and motor blockade.

CURRENT CONTROVERSIES, FUTURE CONSIDERATIONS

Multiple recent studies suggest that the administration of maintenance epidural solutions via PIEB other than CEI may have several benefits for the parturient in labor. Before the re-emergence of data advocating for the use of automated bolus techniques for maintenance of labor analgesia, the use of CEIs with a PCEA, was and may still be the traditional practice in multiple institutions and clinical settings (**Table 1**).

In most studies, PCEA was used as a rescue modality in both the bolus (PIEB) and continuous (CEI) infusion groups. However, PCEA, without a background infusion, is an intermittent bolus technique in itself. Future studies delineating whether the PIEB technique is superior to PCEA when used as the primary mode of analgesic administration would be beneficial.[12] If combination is necessary, automated pumps facilitating the delivery of the combined regimen (timed boluses with PCEA) need to be used during the investigative process since the 2-pump system per parturient used in most studies remains clinically impractical, unrealistic, and cumbersome. Current studies using a single pump to evaluate the efficacy and superiority of the bolus technique with the PCEA (PIEB + PCEA) compared with the CEI + PCEA technique are very limited. One of such studies by Tien and colleagues[7], although retrospective, was unable to replicate significant benefits of the bolus technique compared with the continuous technique. A significant difference among the groups in the ratio of PCEA attempted or given, and the number of unsuccessful PCEA attempts per hour, most likely a surrogate indicator for subject discomfort, was noted. The ratio differences could be an artifact of the increased frequency in which subjects receiving PIEB were locked out from receiving PCEA boluses. Receiving reduced volumes per time period could be a function of frequent lockout periods.[7] Future randomized prospective studies using a single pump, as is the standard clinical practice, need to be performed to address the effect of different flow rates and settings compared with the old pumps and to verify that the outcomes indicated are similar regardless of the pump settings.

Additionally, the benefits of the bolus technique could only be interpreted in the context of the potential differences and variations in the solutions (volume and concentration) used by several studies. As expected, larger boluses of more dilute local anesthetic may improve spread in the epidural space, resulting in better analgesia and, consequently, better patient satisfaction. Also, the use of higher local anesthetic concentration solutions for maintenance of labor, produced a frequent incidence of motor block in both groups. However, according to Fettes and colleagues,[9] the trend was toward less motor block in the PIEB group. Hence, differences between techniques may be driven more by dosing regimens than differences in actual techniques.[5] The need for additional adequately-powered randomized controlled or prospective studies with rigorous controls and standardized drug volume, dose, and concentrations cannot be overstated.[7] The goal is to minimize the mixed results encountered when studying outcome measures such as differences among groups in PCEA requests or administrations, number of manual bolus doses for breakthrough pain, time to first PCEA dose or manual dose, breakthrough pain requiring physician epidural top-up, labor pain scores, motor block, or incidence of instrumental delivery. Although retrospective studies have the advantage of being performed in the real world of clinical care instead of the ideal world of randomized controlled trials, they often depend on the presence of accurate and complete documentation of desired parameters in the electronic medical record. A combination of different types of studies with consistent findings are required.

While it has been shown that increasing bolus volumes and time intervals result in decreased local anesthetic consumption without affecting subject satisfaction, optimal PIEB settings are yet to be determined and confirmed.[7] As noted by Wong and colleagues[10] (2011), the optimal time interval and bolus dose regimen may depend on several factors, including the duration of labor, the concentration and specific components of the epidural solution, and the rate of administration of the programmed bolus dose. Rates of the programmed bolus administration have varied from 75 to 400 mL per hour in several studies.[9,10,13,17–19] The combination of the bolus rate and the epidural catheter tip design may also contribute to the outcome because the infusion or bolus rate influences whether the epidural solution exits 1 or more orifices of a multiorifice catheter.[20] An in vitro study showed that solution exited only the most proximal orifice when the infusion or bolus rate was equal to or less than 120 mL per hour.[20] When the solution is delivered in boluses at higher injection pressure, flow is witnessed through all catheter ports via a multiorifice catheter with greater overall spread. In conjunction with the Wong and colleagues[10] study, additional studies are needed to determine the optimal combination of bolus volume, time interval, and drug combinations for the use of the bolus technique for labor analgesia. Further studies are also necessary to establish whether varying the bolus volumes and intervals are clinically significant and affect important patient clinical outcomes.[10]

With the exception of a few studies that explored the difference in the incidence of instrumental delivery (as a primary endpoint) between both techniques, most studies were designed to examine the efficacy of the bolus technique during the first stage of labor. The study by Capogna and colleagues[1] (2011) was powered to show a difference in motor blockade and the rate of assisted delivery but the use of a more concentrated epidural solution (PCEA) than is often seen in routine clinical practice may have contributed to the higher rate of motor block seen in the CEI group. Differences in instrumental delivery rate may be unlikely with the use of dilute local anesthetic solutions. Additional studies are needed to evaluate the efficacy of the bolus technique compared with the continuous technique during the second stage of labor and for the conversion to operative delivery. Is there a significant difference in the amount of local anesthetic needed to convert labor analgesia to surgical anesthesia based on the maintenance technique used for labor? What are the clinical implications of using 1 technique instead of the other if surgical anesthesia is needed? Is 1 technique likely to mask a patchy, inadequate, epidural block more than the other? What are failure rates of labor epidural catheters in the operative setting based on the maintenance technique used? Although the comparison made in this article is geared toward understanding the optimal epidural maintenance technique for labor analgesia, one cannot ignore the increase in the incidence of operative delivery in the recent years and the idea that a high percentage of labor epidurals will be used for surgical anesthesia for cesarean delivery. More studies need to examine the effect of maintenance techniques in labor on the transition from labor analgesia to surgical anesthesia.

The benefit of decreased local anesthetic consumption with the bolus technique was greater in women with labor of longer duration.[12] Nulliparous women or women undergoing induction of labor may benefit the most. Of note, however, most of the women with clinical indications that would benefit from a decreased amount of local anesthetic and opioid administered for labor analgesia were excluded from the studies. The conclusions made from the various studies are, therefore, limited to the patient population studied and may not be generalizable to all patients encountered in clinical practice. Future studies focusing on maximizing labor analgesia while minimizing maternal and fetal side effects in select challenging patient populations would be beneficial. These select groups include the parturient with congenital (repaired or unrepaired) cardiac disease or hypertensive disorders of pregnancy, systemic disease, morbid obesity, or the use of chronic analgesic medications before pregnancy.

In addition to pregnant women, several other populations use neuraxial analgesia for maintenance of either primary surgical anesthesia or postoperative pain management. Though limited, comparisons of the analgesic effects of PIEB and CEI after other surgical procedures, such as total knee arthroplasty, have been performed. Documented findings have demonstrated a superior analgesic effect, no difference in motor blockade and side effects, and significantly lower rescue medicine usages and numerical rating pain scale for the PIEB group compared with the CEI group.[21] The widespread use of this maintenance technique in the nonobstetric surgical population will create new avenues to explore in the future.

SUMMARY

Documented pain scores have been mostly similar in women receiving CEI or PIEB, hence demonstrating that both techniques can provide excellent labor analgesia in most women. Nonetheless, multiple studies continue to show the PIEB technique as a maintenance mode that offers several other benefits, including the use of less local anesthetic and opioids, the occurrence of less breakthrough pain, the incidence of less motor block subsequently resulting in less instrumental vaginal delivery, and improved patient satisfaction. Most of these studies used the 2-pump system, which is impractical and avoids addressing some of the inherent differences seen when compared with using a single pump, which is routine in clinical practice. The bolus mode of maintaining epidural analgesia may represent a more effective mode of maintenance analgesia for labor. Nevertheless, future prospective adequately powered studies using a single pump under practical conditions are needed to replicate and confirm earlier findings; optimize PIEB and PCEA settings; quantify the ideal desired bolus volumes and time intervals needed within safety limits; refine pump algorithms necessary to ensure that the correct combination of volume, rate, pressures, and frequency of intermittent mandatory boluses and PCEA self-boluses are coupled in tandem; and, most importantly, validate the presence of clinically important improved patient outcomes with this technique.

REFERENCES

1. Capogna G, Camorcia M, Stirparo S, et al. Programmed intermittent epidural bolus versus continuous epidural infusion for labor analgesia: the effects on maternal motor function and labor outcome. A randomized double-blind study in nulliparous women. Anesth Analg 2011;113(4):826–31.
2. Braveman FR, Scavone BM, Wong CA, et al. Obstetrical anesthesia. In: Barash PG, Cullen BF, Stoelting RK, et al, editors. Clinical anesthesia. 6th edition. Philadelphia: Lippincott Williams & Wilkins; 2009. p. 1137–70.
3. Afolabi BB, Lesi FE. Regional versus general anesthesia for caesarean section. Cochrane Database Syst Rev 2012;(10):CD004350.
4. Practice Guidelines for Obstetric Anesthesia: An Updated Report by the American Society of Anesthesiologists Task Force on Obstetric Anesthesia and the Society of Obstetric Anesthesia and Perinatology. Anesthesiology 2016;124(2): 270–300.
5. McKenzie CP, Cobb B, Riley ET, et al. Programmed intermittent epidural boluses for maintenance of labor analgesia: an impact study. Int J Obstet Anesth 2016;26:32–8.
6. Boutros A, Blary S, Bronchard R, et al. Comparison of intermittent epidural bolus, continuous epidural infusion and patient-controlled epidural analgesia during labor. Int J Obstet Anesth 1999;8:236–41.
7. Tien M, Allen TK, Mauritz A, et al. A retrospective comparison of programmed intermittent epidural bolus with continuous epidural infusion using the CADD-Solis v3.0 pump for maintenance of labor analgesia. Curr Med Res Opin 2016; 32(8):1435–40.
8. Capogna G, Stirparo S. Techniques for the maintenance of epidural labor analgesia. Curr Opin Anaesthesiol 2013;26:261–7.
9. Fettes PDW, Moore CS, Whiteside JB, et al. Intermittent vs continuous administration of epidural ropivacaine with fentanyl for analgesia during labour. Br J Anaesth 2006;97(3):359–64.
10. Wong CA, McCarthy RJ, Hewlett B. The effect of manipulation of the programmed intermittent bolus time interval and injection volume on total drug use for labor epidural analgesia: a randomized controlled trial. Anesth Analg 2011;112(4): 904–11.
11. Hogan Q. Distribution of solution in the epidural space: examination by cryomicrotome section. Reg Anesth Pain Med 2002;27:150–6.
12. Wong CA, Ratliff JT, Sullivan JT, et al. A randomized comparison of programmed intermittent epidural bolus with continuous epidural infusion for labor analgesia. Anesth Analg 2006;102:904–9.
13. Leo S, Ocampo Y, Lim Y, et al. A randomized comparison of automated intermittent mandatory boluses with a basal infusion in combination with patient-controlled epidural analgesia for labor and delivery. Int J Obstet Anesth 2010; 19:357–64.
14. Halpern SH, Carvalho B. Patient-controlled epidural analgesia for labor. Anesth Analg 2009;108(3):921–8.

15. Sezer OA, Gunaydin B. Efficacy of patient-controlled epidural analgesia after initiation with epidural or combined spinal-epidural analgesia. Int J Obstet Anesth 2007;16:226–30.
16. George RB, Allen TK, Habib AS. Intermittent epidural bolus compared with continuous epidural infusions for labor analgesia: review and meta-analysis. Anesth Analg 2013;116(1):133–44.
17. Lim Y, Chakravarty S, Ocampo CE, et al. Comparison of automated intermittent low volume bolus with continuous infusion for labour epidural analgesia. Anaesth Intensive Care 2010;38:894–9.
18. Sia AT, Lim Y, Ocampo C. A comparison of basal infusion with automated mandatory boluses in parturient-controlled epidural analgesia during labor. Anesth Analg 2007,104.073–8.
19. Chua OM, Sia AT. Automated intermittent epidural boluses improve analgesia induced by intrathecal fentanyl during labour. Can J Anaesth 2004;51:581–5.
20. Fegley AJ, Lerman J, Wissler R. Epidural multiorifice catheters function as a single-orifice catheters: an in vitro study. Anesth Analg 2008;107:1079–81.
21. Kang S, Jeon S, Choe JH, et al. Comparison of analgesic effects of programmed intermittent epidural bolus and continuous epidural infusion after total knee arthroplasty. Korean J Anesthesiol 2013;65(6 Suppl):S130–1 (Letter to the Editor).

Identification and Management of Obstetric Hemorrhage

Emily J. Baird, MD, PhD

KEYWORDS

- Obstetric hemorrhage • Uterine atony • Transfusion • Fibrinogen
- Recombinant activated factor VII • Tranexamic acid • Cell salvage

KEY POINTS

- Prevention of adverse outcomes in obstetric hemorrhage depends on stepwise, escalating interventions, including pharmacologic, hematological, radiological, and surgical interventions.
- Timely red blood cell transfusion is critical in the maintenance of adequate intravascular volume, tissue oxygenation, and effective coagulation.
- Given the significant risk of coagulopathy with massive bleeding, fresh frozen plasma should be considered early in the resuscitation of obstetric hemorrhage.
- Fibrinogen may play a unique role in the diagnosis and management of obstetric hemorrhage.
- Intraoperative cell salvage techniques decrease transfusion requirements with minimal additional risk.

INTRODUCTION

Obstetric hemorrhage remains the leading cause of maternal death and severe morbidity worldwide. In developing nations, including Africa and Asia, peripartum hemorrhage is responsible for 30% of all direct maternal mortality.[1] Despite advances in obstetric and transfusion medicine, well-resourced countries are not impervious to this potentially catastrophic complication, with peripartum bleeding accounting for 3.4% and 11.8% of maternal deaths in the United Kingdom and United States, respectively.[2,3] Significant morbidity, in the form of loss of fertility, pituitary necrosis, renal insufficiency, coagulopathy, and respiratory failure, is also associated with severe peripartum bleeding.[4] Although uterine atony is the most common cause of hemorrhage, abnormal placentation, coagulation disorders, and genital tract trauma also contribute to significant morbidity and mortality. Despite the identification of many

Department of Anesthesiology and Perioperative Medicine, Oregon Health and Science University, 3181 Southwest Sam Jackson Park Road, Mailcode UH2, Portland, OR 97239, USA
E-mail address: Bairde@ohsu.edu

Anesthesiology Clin 35 (2017) 15–34
http://dx.doi.org/10.1016/j.anclin.2016.09.004   **anesthesiology.theclinics.com**

characteristics associated with obstetric hemorrhage, most parturients who subsequently experience significant bleeding have no recognizable risk factors. Given the inability to reliably predict patients at high risk for obstetric hemorrhage, all parturients should be considered susceptible, and extreme vigilance must be exercised in the assessment of blood loss and hemodynamic stability during the peripartum period. Obstetric-specific hemorrhage protocols, facilitating the integration and timely escalation of pharmacologic, radiological, surgical, and transfusion interventions, are critical to the successful management of peripartum bleeding.

DEFINITION OF OBSTETRIC HEMORRHAGE

The precise definition of obstetric hemorrhage remains nebulous, with numerous classification systems currently in use worldwide (Box 1).[5–7] Given the dynamic changes in plasma volume commonly accompanying the peripartum period, the use of acute changes in hematocrit (Hct) is of limited utility in the timely diagnosis of significant bleeding. Most international guidelines rely on estimation of blood loss and/or hemodynamic instability to identify peripartum hemorrhage. In the United States, blood loss

---

Box 1
Summary of international obstetric hemorrhage definitions currently in use

American Congress of Obstetricians and Gynecologists Guidelines
- "No single, satisfactory definition[6]
- Conventional definition:
  - Blood loss greater than 500 mL following vaginal delivery
  - Blood loss greater than 1000 mL following cesarean delivery

Australian Guidelines
- Blood loss greater than 500 mL following vaginal delivery
- Blood loss greater than 750 mL following cesarean delivery

Austrian Society of Obstetrics and Gynaecology[6]
- Blood loss 500 to 1000 mL with clinical signs of hypovolemic shock
- Blood loss greater than 1000 mL

German Society of Obstetrics and Gynaecology[6]
- Blood loss greater than 500 mL following vaginal delivery
- Blood loss greater than 1000 mL following cesarean delivery

Royal College of Obstetricians and Gynaecologists[6]
- Blood loss 500 to 1000 mL
- *Severe* obstetric hemorrhage
  - Blood loss greater than 1000 mL
  - Blood loss 500 to 1000 mL with clinical signs of hypovolemic shock

World Health Organization[5]
- Blood loss greater than 500 mL
- *Severe* obstetric hemorrhage
  - Blood loss greater than 1000 mL

Adapted from Rath WH. Postpartum hemorrhage—update on problems of definitions and diagnosis. Acta Obstet Gynecol Scand 2011;90(5):421–8.

exceeding 500 mL for vaginal delivery and 1000 mL for cesarean delivery has traditionally been used in the classification of obstetric hemorrhage. These values are of questionable clinical significance given that they are only slightly higher than the average blood loss for each mode of delivery. Furthermore, the expansion of blood volume typically accompanying pregnancy confers a protective advantage, and blood losses of 1000 mL are generally well tolerated. Recently, an international panel of experts in the fields of obstetrics, gynecology, hematology, and anesthesiology proposed the following diagnostic criteria for the identification of women at increased risk of adverse outcomes from obstetric hemorrhage:

> *Active bleeding > 1000 mL within the 24 hours following birth that continues despite the use of initial measures, including first-line uterotonic agents and uterine massage.*[5]

Although a unified definition will facilitate comparison of the incidence and outcomes of obstetric hemorrhage among different countries, the clinical significance of 1000 mL of blood loss in 24 hours is questionable.

CAUSES OF OBSTETRIC HEMORRHAGE

Obstetric hemorrhage is an all-inclusive term referring to several distinct pathways ultimately resulting in significant peripartum blood loss. Causes of obstetric hemorrhage have traditionally been classified as "antepartum" or "postpartum," in reference to the timing of maternal bleeding in relation to the delivery of the fetus (**Box 2**). The presence of coagulation disorders, both congenital and acquired, can further contribute to the incidence and severity of obstetric hemorrhage. An understanding of the unique mechanisms, risk factors, and clinical manifestations of these distinct causes of peripartum bleeding is critical in the early identification and successful management of obstetric hemorrhage.

Box 2
Common causes of and/or contributors to obstetric hemorrhage

Antepartum Hemorrhage

- Placenta previa
- Uterine rupture
- Placental abruption

Postpartum Hemorrhage

- Uterine atony
- Placenta accreta
- Genital trauma

Congenital Coagulation Disorders

- von Willebrand disease
- Hemophilia A
- Hemophilia B
- Glanzmann thrombasthenia
- Bernard-Soulier syndrome

Antepartum Obstetric Hemorrhage

Placenta previa

Placenta previa, complicating 1 in 200 pregnancies, is characterized by the presence of the placenta overlying the endocervical os (**Fig. 1**).[8,9] Risk factors include previous uterine surgery and a history of placenta previa.[10,11] Disruption of the placental attachment from the uterine decidua can lead to significant bleeding and uteroplacental insufficiency. The classic presentation is "painless vaginal bleeding," but abdominal pain and/or contractions may also occur.[10] Diagnosis is confirmed with the use transabdominal and/or transvaginal ultrasound to delineate the relationship of placenta to the endocervical os. Placenta previa is an indication for cesarean delivery.

Uterine rupture

Uterine rupture, defined as a full-thickness separation of the uterine wall and the overlying serosa, occurs in approximately 1 in 100 parturients with a prior uterine surgery.[12,13] Factors compromising the integrity of the uterine wall, including grand multiparity, fetal malpresentation, and oxytocin augmentation of labor, can further increase the risk of uterine rupture.[14] Clinical manifestations include a non-reassuring fetal heart rate, abdominal pain, hypotension, cessation of labor, and palpation of fetal parts in the abdomen. Urgent cesarean delivery is indicated.

Placental abruption

Placental abruption develops in 1 in 150 pregnancies.[15,16] Antepartum separation of the placenta from the decidua basalis may lead to significant blood loss and compromised placental blood flow. Hypertension, preeclampsia, cocaine use, tobacco use, and abdominal trauma have been associated with an increased risk of placenta abruption.[17] Classic findings include painful vaginal bleeding, abdominal tenderness, and irritable uterine contraction pattern.[17] Delivery is generally indicated unless the fetus is premature *and* the abruption is small with minimal maternal and fetal hemodynamic sequela.

Postpartum Obstetric Hemorrhage

Uterine atony

Uterine atony is responsible for approximately 80% of postpartum hemorrhages.[4] At term gestation, blood flow to the uterus is approximately 700 mL/min. Following

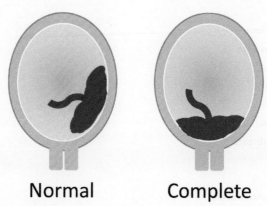

Normal   Complete

Fig. 1. Placenta previa describes a condition whereby the placenta partially or completely covers the cervix.

placental delivery, contraction of the uterus leads to compression of the spiral arteries supplying the placental bed. Inadequate myometrial tone allows continued maternal perfusion of the unoccupied placental bed, resulting in significant postpartum blood loss. Several antepartum characteristics have been associated with the subsequent development of uterine atony (**Box 3**).[18] Unfortunately, predicting the occurrence of postpartum hemorrhage is challenging given that less than 40% of parturients with uterine atony resulting in transfusion had an identifiable risk factor.[4] Management of uterine atony involves administration of uterotonic agents (discussed later), uterine massage, and manual removal of retained placental tissue. Invasive methods for controlling blood loss associated with uterine atony unresponsive to more conservation measures include the Bakri balloon, B-Lynch compression sutures, and hysterectomy (discussed later).

Placenta accreta

Accreta refers to a spectrum of abnormal placentation, characterized by the aberrant attachment of the placenta to the uterus. Placenta accreta is further classified based on the depth of placental uterine invasion (**Fig. 2**). Placenta accreta vera describes placental attachment directly to the myometrium, without an intervening decidua basalis layer. Placental infiltration *into* the uterine myometrium is designated increta, whereas percreta describes placental invasion *through* the uterine serosa, and potentially into surrounding pelvic structures. Regardless of the degree of uterine invasion, all variations of placenta accreta are associated with postpartum hemorrhage given the significant challenge in removing the placenta following delivery.

The incidence of placenta accreta has risen exponentially over the past 50 years, with recent estimates suggesting a rate of approximately 1 in 500 pregnancies.[19] The increased occurrence of abnormal placentation parallels the increase in invasive maternal obstetric and gynecologic interventions, including cesarean delivery, uterine embolization, and myomectomy. Because placenta accreta is generally asymptomatic before delivery, antenatal diagnosis is dependent on noninvasive imaging techniques. When performed by an experienced sonographer, ultrasound combined with color Doppler has a diagnostic sensitivity, specificity, and negative predictive value of approximately 80%, 90%, and 98%, respectively.[20,21] Ultrasound findings

---

Box 3
Conditions associated with uterine atony

Uterine distension
- High parity
- Multiple gestations
- Polyhydramnios
- Macrosomia

Oxytocin desensitization
- Induced or prolonged labor

Impaired uterine involution
- Retained placenta
- Placenta accreta

Decreased myometrial tone
- Volatile halogenated anesthetic agents
- Magnesium
- Tocolytic agents

Chorioamnionitis

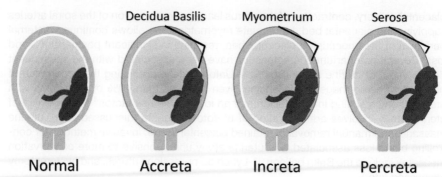

Decidua Basilis   Myometrium   Serosa

Normal   Accreta   Increta   Percreta

Fig. 2. Placenta accrete occurs when all or part of the placenta attaches abnormally to the myometrium. The 3 grades of abnormal placental attachment are defined according to the depth of uterine invasion.

suggestive of placenta accreta include loss of the normal retroplacental-myometrial hypoechoic zone, increased vascularity within the uterine wall, and the presence of multiple vascular lacunae (creating a "moth-eaten or Swiss cheese" appearance).[20,21] Early identification of placenta accreta facilitates the coordination of multidisciplinary postpartum management, which frequently involves massive transfusion in conjunction with a combined cesarean delivery–hysterectomy.

Genital trauma
Vaginal delivery is associated with varying degrees of injury to the vagina, vulva, and/or cervix. Risk factors associated with lower genital tract trauma during childbirth include nulliparity, macrosomia, precipitous delivery, forceps- or vacuum-assisted delivery, and/or episiotomy.[15,22] Although cervical laceration complicates 50% of vaginal deliveries,[23] most injuries are superficial with minimal hematologic consequences. Lacerations extending into the lower uterine segment, uterine artery, and/or retroperitoneum can be associated with significant blood loss and hemodynamic perturbations, requiring pharmacologic, hematological, and/or surgical intervention.

Coagulation Disorders
Pregnancy is characterized as a hypercoagulable state, with an increase in many coagulation factors and a decrease in the activity of anticoagulant and fibrinolytic pathways (**Fig. 3**).[24] Inherited coagulation disorders can disrupt these protective prohemostatic changes. Parturients with hereditary hematologic disorders, most frequently von Willebrand disease, hemophilia, and platelet disorders, are at an increased risk of significant obstetric bleeding. Recommendations for the prophylactic treatment of parturients with inherited bleeding disorders are included in **Table 1**.[5]

MANAGEMENT OF OBSTETRIC HEMORRHAGE
Obstetric Hemorrhage Protocol

Most fatalities associated with obstetric hemorrhage are preventable, with "substandard care" contributing to approximately 70% of maternal mortality.[25–27] Adverse outcomes have been attributed to several avoidable factors, including underestimation of blood loss, lack of blood product availability, insufficient interdisciplinary communication, and delayed escalation of invasive interventions.[25] Obstetric-specific massive transfusion algorithms have been associated with a decrease in maternal morbidity.[28] Despite the proven success of obstetric hemorrhage protocols, a recent survey

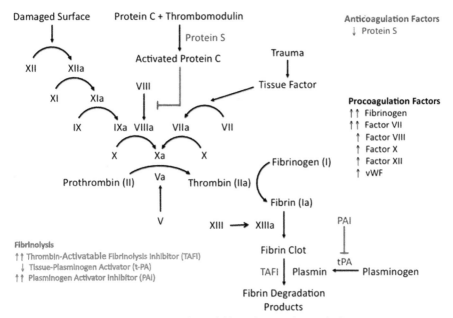

Fig. 3. Changes in coagulation cascade and fibrinolytic pathway during pregnancy.

Table 1
Recommendations for the prophylactic treatment of women with inherited bleeding disorders

Coagulation Disorder	Characteristics	Management
von Willebrand disease		
Type 1	vWF deficiency	TXA, DDAVP
Type 2	vWF dysfunction	TXA, vWF concentrates
Type 3	vWF absent	TXA, vWF concentrates
Hypofibrinogenemia	Fibrinogen deficiency	Fibrinogen concentrate, cryoprecipitate, FFP
Dysfibrinogenemia	Fibrinogen dysfunction	Treatment individualized based on risk of bleeding vs thrombosis
FII	Factor II deficiency	PCC
FV	Factor V deficiency	FFP
FVII	Factor VII deficiency	rFVIIa
Hemophilia A	Factor VIII deficiency	TXA, DDAVP, FVIII replacement
Hemophilia B	Factor IX deficiency	TXA, Factor IX replacement
FX	Factor X deficiency	FX concentrate, PCC
Glanzmann thrombasthenia	Platelet dysfunction	TXA, Factor VIIa, platelets
Bernard-Soulier syndrome	Platelet dysfunction and deficiency	TXA, Factor VIIa, platelets

Abbreviations: DDAVP, desmopression; PCC, prothrombin complex concentrate.

Adapted from Abdul-Kadir R, McLintock C, Ducloy AS, et al. Evaluation and management of postpartum hemorrhage: consensus from an international expert panel. Transfusion 2014;54(7):1756–68; with permission.

suggested that they are in practice in less than 70% of labor and delivery units within the United States.[29] In response to the alarming increase in obstetric hemorrhage and associated morbidity and mortality, the National Partnership for Maternal Safety (NPMS) has developed a safety bundle, outlining critical clinical practices that should be implemented in every maternity unit (**Box 4**).[30] The obstetric safety bundle emphasizes the basic tenets of crisis management, namely readiness, recognition and prevention, response, and reporting and systems learning. Application of obstetric-specific protocols, facilitating the integration and timely escalation of pharmacologic, radiological, surgical, and transfusion interventions, is critical to reducing maternal morbidity and mortality associated with peripartum bleeding. Successful implementation of the NPMS recommendations requires multidisciplinary collaboration, ongoing resource assessment and allocation, unwavering provider vigilance, and a commitment to system processes improvement. Although initial application and continued maintenance of the NPMS recommendations require an investment of both personnel and financial resources, it will unquestionably contribute to improve maternal outcomes in the setting of obstetric hemorrhage.

Box 4
Obstetric hemorrhage safety bundle from the National Partnership for Maternal Safety, Council on Patient Safety in Women's Health Care

Readiness (Every Unit)

- Hemorrhage cart with supplies, checklist, and instruction cards for intrauterine balloons and compression stitches
- Immediate access to hemorrhage medications (kit or equivalent)
- Establish a response team: who to call when help is needed (blood bank, advanced gynecologic surgery, other support and tertiary services)
- Establish massive and emergency-release transfusion protocols (type O–negative or un-cross-matched RBC, FFP, platelets, cryoprecipitate)
- Unit education or protocols, unit-based drills (with post–drill debriefs)

Recognition and Prevention (Every Patient)

- Assessment of hemorrhage risk (prenatal, intrapartum, postpartum)
- Measurement of cumulative blood loss (formal, as quantitative as possible)
- Active management of the third stage of labor (department-wide protocol)

Response (Every Hemorrhage)

- Unit-standard, stage-based obstetric hemorrhage emergency management plan with checklists
- Support program for patients, families, and staff for all significant hemorrhage

Reporting and Systems Learning (Every Unit)

- Establish a culture of huddles for high-risk patients and postevent debriefs to identify successes and opportunities
- Multidisciplinary review of serious hemorrhages for systems issues
- Monitor outcomes and process metrics in perinatal quality improvement committee

Adapted from Main EK, Goffman D, Scavone BM, et al. National partnership for maternal safety: consensus bundle on obstetric hemorrhage. Anesth Analg 2015;121(1):142–8; with permission.

Estimation of Blood Loss

The most common trigger for initiation of obstetric hemorrhage protocols is blood loss exceeding 1500 mL. Timely identification of hemorrhage is complicated by inherent inaccuracies in visual estimation of blood loss and the lack of early hemodynamic changes. Several studies have indicated that visual assessment of blood loss is grossly unreliable, with actual losses frequently exceeding twice the reported visual estimations.[31] Physiologic perturbations are often late signs of hypovolemia in young, healthy parturients (**Table 2**). Peripheral and splanchnic vasoconstriction facilitates the relocation of blood from venous capacitance vessels to the central circulation, allowing the blood pressure and heart rate to remain near normal until blood loss exceeds 1500 mL in most parturients. Laboratory evaluation is generally too slow to meaningfully reflect dynamic changes in Hct and coagulation status during an obstetric hemorrhage. Precision in blood loss assessment is improved with the use of widely available pictorial guidelines and/or meticulous physical collection systems.[32] Given the challenges in the accurate estimation of blood loss during delivery, extreme vigilance is necessary to assure the early recognition and treatment of obstetric hemorrhage.

Pharmacologic Treatment

Because uterine atony is the primary cause of obstetric hemorrhage, the early administration of uterotonic agents should be considered in the setting of significant postpartum bleeding. Uterotonic medications decrease blood loss by directly stimulating uterine contractions, thus compressing the spiral arteries supplying the vacant placental bed. Oxytocin is generally regarded as the "first-line" pharmacologic intervention for postpartum hemorrhage. Previous studies have demonstrated that prophylactic use of oxytocin during the third stage of labor decreases the incidence of obstetric hemorrhage.[33] Other classes of uterotonic agents should be considered if uterine atony is unresponsive to oxytocin. The specific "second-line" pharmacologic intervention is dependent on the presence of maternal comorbidities. Administration guidelines and contraindications of commonly used uterotonic agents are included in **Table 3**.

Invasive Obstetric Management

Obstetric hemorrhage unresponsive to uterotonic agents may require mechanical or surgical interventions to control blood loss. Uterine massage stimulates myometrial contractions, although the benefit in the setting of ongoing uterotonic administration is questionable.[34,35] Internal uterine tamponade decreases blood loss by compressing

Table 2
Signs and symptoms of blood loss with obstetric hemorrhage in the healthy parturient

Blood Loss (mL)	Systolic Blood Pressure (mm Hg)	Heart Rate (bpm)	Symptoms
1000	>100	<100	Palpitations, lightheadedness
1500	90–100	100–120	Weakness, diaphoresis
2000	70–80	120–140	Restlessness, confusion, pallor
3000	50–70	>140	Lethargy, air hunger

Adapted from Bonnar J. Massive obstetric haemorrhage. Baillieres Best Pract Res Clin Obstet Gynaecol 2000;14(1):1–18.

Table 3
Medications for uterine atony

Uterotonic Agent	Route/Dose	Frequency	Contraindications	Side Effects
Oxytocin (Pitocin)	Intravenous (IV): 10–40 U/L	Infusion	None	Hypotension
	Intramuscular (IM): 10 U	Once		Nausea/vomiting Free water retention
Methylergonovine (Methergin)	IM: 0.2 mg	Every 2–4 h	Hypertension Coronary disease Raynaud	Nausea/vomiting Hypertension
15-methyl PGF$_{2\alpha}$ (Hemabate, Carboprost)	IM: 0.25 mg	Every 15–90 min (8 doses maximum)	Reactive airway Pulmonary hypertension	Bronchoconstriction Shivering Diarrhea ↑ Temperature
Misoprostol (Cytotec)	Buccal: 400 µg Rectal: 1000 µg	Once Once	None	Nausea/vomiting Shivering Diarrhea ↑ Temperature

intrauterine vessels and bleeding surfaces. Intrauterine placement of a Foley catheter or Bakri balloon allows simultaneous compression of uterine surfaces with cavity drainage for monitoring of ongoing blood loss (**Fig. 4**). External uterine compression can be accomplished with the use of circumferential (B-Lynch) uterine sutures (**Fig. 5**). Retrospective studies have demonstrated decreases in blood loss and postpartum hysterectomy rates with the use of internal uterine tamponade and/or external compression sutures in the setting of obstetric hemorrhage.[36] Blood flow to the uterus can be restricted further with surgical ligation or embolization of the uterine arteries. When escalating mechanical and fertility-preserving surgical/radiological interventions are ineffective, hysterectomy should be considered for the definitive management of obstetric hemorrhage.

Resuscitation

There is currently no consensus on the optimal pathway for resuscitation of massive bleeding in the obstetric patient. Given the unique changes in the coagulation and

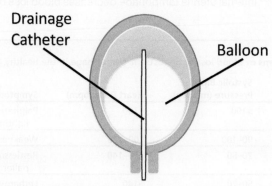

Fig. 4. Intrauterine balloon tamponade exerts pressure against the uterine wall to reduce venous bleeding from the endometrium and myometrium. A central drainage catheter helps quantitate ongoing uterine bleeding.

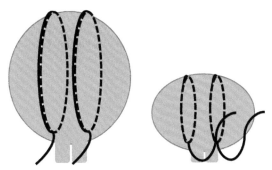

Fig. 5. B-Lynch sutures are used to mechanically compress an atonic uterus in the setting of severe postpartum hemorrhage.

fibrinolytic systems accompanying pregnancy, most obstetric-specific massive transfusion protocols suggest resuscitation with the early administration of red blood cells (RBC), fresh frozen plasma (FFP), cryoprecipitate, and platelets. In the setting of hemorrhage unresponsive to blood component therapy, consideration should be given to prohemostatic and antifibrinolytic agents. Furthermore, the use of cell salvage techniques offers the ability to recycle blood lost from the surgical field, potentially minimizing heterologous transfusion and associated complications.

Crystalloid and colloids

Rapid restoration of intravascular volume is generally initiated with the use of warmed, non-dextrose-containing crystalloid, including lactated Ringer solution and normal saline. Crystalloid is typically administered in a ratio of 3:1 in relation to estimated blood loss. Although crystalloid is useful for initial resuscitation and/or mild hemorrhage, previous studies have demonstrated that only 20% of the crystalloid volume remains intravascular an hour after infusion.[15] Re-equilibration of large crystalloid volumes can lead to interstitial edema and impairment of microcirculation.

Given the transient intravascular effect of crystalloid resuscitation, volume expansion with synthetic colloid solutions had been previously proposed. Although synthetic colloids are effective in prolonged restoration of circulating volume, they have been associated with inhibition of platelet aggregation, impaired clot formation, and increased blood loss.[37,38] Furthermore, recent studies in nonpregnant patients have demonstrated that colloid resuscitation is associated with a significant increase in cost but no benefit in outcomes.[39,40] Synthetic colloid administration is therefore *not* indicated in the management of obstetric hemorrhage.

Red blood cells

Although crystalloid can restore intravascular volume, RBC are needed to ensure adequate oxygen-carrying capacity of blood and avoid acidosis. The transfusion of 1 unit of RBC is expected to increase the Hct by 3% to 5%.[15] The threshold at which RBC replacement should be initiated depends on the presence of comorbidities, hemodynamic parameters, and anticipated additional blood loss. Although an Hct of 18% to 25% may be well tolerated in an otherwise healthy parturient, most experts agree that RBC transfusion is warranted with a Hct less than 25% in the setting of ongoing hemorrhage.[15] A higher Hct during active bleeding not only maintains tissue and organ perfusion but also improves overall coagulation.[41]

Coagulation involves the intimate interplay between RBC, plasma coagulation factors, platelets, and the endothelium. Adequate RBC mass is essential in coordinating the interactions between platelets and the vessel wall. A reduction in RBC mass (anemia) leads to marked decreases in both blood viscosity and resistance to blood flow. The resulting fast transit of platelets through central luminal flow causes a reduction in crucial platelet and endothelial cell interactions necessary for primary hemostasis. Timely RBC transfusion is critical in the maintenance of adequate intravascular volume, tissue oxygenation, and effective coagulation.

Fresh frozen plasma

The development of an acquired coagulopathy, from consumptive and dilutional effects, frequently complicates obstetric hemorrhage. Although pregnancy is associated with an increase in procoagulant activity and a decrease in fibrinolytic pathways, these protective mechanisms are overwhelmed in the setting of massive blood loss. Effective hemostasis is generally maintained if the concentration of coagulation factors does not decrease beyond 30% of normal levels. The brisk bleeding characteristic of obstetric hemorrhage can lead to the rapid consumption of clotting proteins and platelets, exceeding the normal surplus of coagulation factors. Critical levels of prothrombin, factor V (FV), FVII, and platelets are reached after a loss of greater than 200% of calculated blood volume, whereas life threatening levels of fibrinogen are reached after a loss of only 140%.[42] Aggressive replacement of intravascular volume with crystalloid and RBC can lead to dilution of coagulation factors and platelets, further impeding hemostatic mechanisms.

The prompt implementation of prohemostatic interventions is critical in preventing complications from uncontrolled coagulopathy. Each unit of FFP increases coagulation factor levels by approximately 8%.[43] Although traditional guidelines suggest FFP should be used only in the setting of an elevated prothrombin time or activated partial thromboplastin time, recent data emerging from the trauma and obstetric literature endorse a more aggressive repletion of coagulation factors. The trauma literature suggests 1:1 FFP:RBC resuscitation ratio is associated with faster reversal of coagulopathy, decreased blood loss, and lower mortality.[44] Although the parturient population is distinctly different from that encountered in military and civilian trauma, preliminary obstetric hemorrhage research corroborate the findings of improved outcomes with more aggressive procoagulant transfusion strategies.[45] A recent, large retrospective study of transfusion in postpartum hemorrhage found an association between a higher FFP:RBC ratio and lower odds of requiring an advanced interventional procedure, including uterine artery embolization and/or hysterectomy.[45] Given the significant risk of coagulopathy with massive bleeding, FFP should be considered early in the resuscitation of obstetric hemorrhage.

Fibrinogen

Fibrinogen, the final factor in the coagulation cascade, may play a unique role in the diagnosis and management of obstetric hemorrhage. Fibrinogen concentration substantially increases during the third trimester, with term parturients having fibrinogen levels of approximately 4.5 to 5.8 g/L compared with nonpregnant control levels of 2.0 to 4.5 g/L.[46] Several studies have identified decreased fibrinogen levels as an important predictor of severe obstetric hemorrhage.[47–49] Charbit and colleagues[47] reported the risk of severe postpartum bleeding increased by a factor of 2.6 for each 1 g/L decrease in fibrinogen level. Baseline plasma fibrinogen level less than 2 g/L at the time of bleeding onset had a positive predictive value of 100% for subsequent evolution to severe hemorrhage, whereas plasma fibrinogen level greater than 4 g/L had a 79% negative predictive value for significant blood loss.[47] It is unclear whether decreased fibrinogen levels simply reflect the severity of blood loss or if it is an independent and measurable risk factor that could potentially be used as a diagnostic tool in the early identification of obstetric hemorrhage.

Given the correlation between hypofibrinogenemia and severe obstetric bleeding, fibrinogen has emerged as a potential therapeutic target for the management of postpartum hemorrhage. Fibrinogen, which is essential for clot strength and speed of clot formation, is one of the first coagulation factors to decrease beyond critical levels during massive blood loss.[46,50] Although transfusion guidelines historically recommended fibrinogen replacement with levels less than 1 g/L, a recent in vitro study suggests that fibrinogen levels of 2.5 g/L are associated with optimal clot formation.[42] The elevated levels of fibrinogen in pregnancy and the observed progression to severe bleeding in parturients with levels less than 2 g/L further support the maintenance of higher fibrinogen concentrations.[5] In addition, the rapid restoration of normal peripartum fibrinogen levels (4–6 g/L) has been shown to effectively reduce or arrest blood loss.[51–53]

Although FFP, cryoprecipitate, and fibrinogen concentrates can all be used to increase fibrinogen levels, the optimal strategy for managing hypofibrinogenemia in obstetric hemorrhage is unclear. The relatively low concentration of fibrinogen in FFP limits its usefulness in the treatment of significant hypofibrinogenemia.[54] To increase fibrinogen plasma level by 1 g/L, 30 mL/kg of FFP is necessary, increasing the risk of pulmonary edema and other hypervolemic complications.[55] Cryoprecipitate, which is a concentrated source of fibrinogen, factor VIII, fibronectin, von Willebrand factor (vWF), and factor XIII, will increase fibrinogen levels by ~0.7 to 1 g/L for every 100 mL given.[56] Although cryoprecipitate is associated with a lower transfusion volume, the standard "dose" (10 U) is typically prepared by pooling concentrates from multiple donors.[29] Given the risk of infectious disease transmission and/or an immunologic reaction from exposure to multiple donors, several countries preferentially use purified, pasteurized fibrinogen concentrate for the treatment of congenital and/or acquired hypofibrinogenemia. Fibrinogen concentrates are also prepared from large donor pools, but subsequent processing removes or inactivates potentially contaminating viruses, antibodies, and antigens. Studies comparing cryoprecipitate and fibrinogen concentrates utilization in hemorrhage resuscitation suggest fibrinogen concentrates are associated with lower blood loss, decreased RBC transfusion, and greater increases in plasma fibrinogen levels.[51,57] Although the most appropriate method of fibrinogen replacement is somewhat controversial, the critical role of fibrinogen in reversing the coagulopathy accompanying obstetric hemorrhage is clear. As such, close monitoring and replacement of fibrinogen are crucial in the management of the bleeding parturient.

Platelets

Platelets are another essential component of coagulation, with quantitative and qualitative platelet deficiencies contributing to inadequate hemostasis. Fibrinogen degradation products and anemia are commonly associated with obstetric hemorrhage and can inhibit platelet function. Initial resuscitation with crystalloid, RBC, and FFP can lead to a dilutional thrombocytopenia, further impeding adequate platelet activity. A platelet count of at least 50,000/mm^3 should be maintained in the setting of active bleeding to optimize adequate clot formation. One unit of platelets, which is typically compiled from 6 donors, will generally increase levels by 25,000 to 30,000/mm^3.[29] Although not required, ABO compatibility increases the lifespan of transfused platelets. Of note, rhesus (Rh) sensitivity can occur in an Rh-negative recipient due to the presence of a few red cells in Rh-positive unit.

Procoagulation Agents

In the setting of intractable obstetric hemorrhage, procoagulation agent recombinant activated factor VII (rFVIIa) may be considered. rFVIIa is a synthetic vitamin K–dependent glycoprotein that aids in hemostasis via activation of the extrinsic pathway of the coagulation cascade.[58] Although currently approved only for use in hemophilia, factor VII deficiency, and Glanzmann thrombasthenia, several groups have reported the successful treatment of obstetric hemorrhage with rFVIIa. Retrospective studies investigating the use of rFVIIa in the management of obstetric hemorrhage unresponsive to conventional therapies have suggested rFVIIa is associated with decreased blood loss, reduced RBC transfusion, and lower maternal mortality.[59–61] Although preliminary reports are certainly encouraging, there is some concern that use of rFVIIa may contribute to subsequent thrombotic complications.[62] Given the paucity of randomized controlled trials (RCTs) to unequivocally define the efficacy and safety profile of its administration, rFVIIa should be used only after failure of conventional therapies, including invasive treatment (such as uterine embolization) but before obstetric hysterectomy.

The effectiveness of rFVIIa depends on an optimal hemostatic environment. rFVIIa is an enzyme, with temperature, acid-base status (pH), and substrate availability significantly influencing its function. Previous studies have demonstrated rFVIIa is maximally effective when the following parameters are achieved: temperature greater than 34°C, arterial pH greater than 7.20, normocalcemia, Hct greater than 30%, platelet count greater than 50,000/mm^3, and fibrinogen greater than 1 g/L.[41] Although the optimal rFVIIa dose for the parturient is not well defined, 60 to 90 μg/kg is commonly used. Given the short half-life of rFVIIa (2 hours), the dose may be repeated within 30 to 60 minutes if there is insufficient improvement in hemostasis and ongoing nonarterial bleeding.[41]

Antifibrinolytic Therapy

Antifibrinolytics, which inhibit the enzymatic degradation of fibrin clots, may play a unique role in the prophylaxis against and management of obstetric hemorrhage. Although fibrinolytic capacity decreases during the last trimester of pregnancy, fibrinolysis increases in the postpartum period.[63] Tranexamic acid (TXA) is a potent antifibrinolytic agent that exerts its effects by blocking lysine binding sites on plasminogen molecules, inhibiting the activation of plasmin. TXA in nonobstetric populations has shown a significant reduction in perioperative blood loss and RBC transfusion without an increase in thrombotic events.[64–66] Studies exploring antifibrinolytic treatment of menorrhagia suggest that TXA can reduce nonsurgical, low-volume, uterine blood loss.[67] Several small RCTs and meta-analyses investigating TXA use in the postpartum period demonstrate that antifibrinolytic therapy is associated with a reduction in blood loss, decreased need for additional uterotonic agents, and higher hemoglobin levels at 24 hours.[68–72] There is currently no consensus on the optimal dosing or timing of TXA administration. In addition, further studies addressing neonatal safety are indicated given that TXA crosses the placenta.[73] It is hoped that a large, randomized, double-blind controlled trial, the World Maternal Antifibrinolytic Trial (WOMAN), currently underway in Europe and Africa, will provide insight into the efficacy and safety of TXA in the prevention and/or treatment of obstetric hemorrhage.[74] The WOMAN trial is designed to measure the effect of early TXA administration on maternal outcomes, including blood transfusion, surgical intervention, nonfatal vascular events, hysterectomy, and death.

Cell Salvage

Intraoperative blood salvage techniques decrease transfusion requirements with minimal additional risk. Blood collected from the surgical field is centrifuged, washed, and filtered to yield RBC with a high Hct (60%–80%). The favorable physiologic profile, including pH, morphology, osmotic stability, and 2,3 diphosphoglycerate content, contribute to increased oxygen carrying capacity and survival of salvaged blood compared with its stored counterpart.[75] Furthermore, use of recycled, autologous blood minimizes the risk of alloimmunization, viral transmission, and hemolytic transfusion reactions. Because processing of scavenged blood removes platelets and activated clotting factors, a dilutional coagulopathy can develop with exclusive transfusion of salvaged blood. In addition, bacterial contamination can complicate processing, although there are no reports of sepsis or infection with the use of cell salvage.[76,77] Finally, administration of salvaged blood through a leukocyte depletion filter can (rarely) lead to disruption of leukocytes with release of cytokines and transient hypotension.[75] Given the nominal risk of adverse effects and the potential to significantly reduce heterologous transfusion requirements, cell salvage techniques are increasingly used for operative procedures.

Although the benefits of intraoperative blood salvage in nonobstetric surgery are well established, universal acceptance of this technique in parturients has been plagued by concerns over amniotic fluid embolism (AFE) and induction of maternal alloimmunization. AFE is an anaphylactoid syndrome presumed to be caused by an unknown fetal antigen.[75] Leukocyte depletion filters have been shown to reduce levels of fetal contaminants, such as lamellar bodies, phospholipids, squamous cells, and amniotic fluid–derived tissue factor, with postwashed, postfiltered salvaged blood containing similar levels of impurities to that found in the maternal circulation.[78,79] A retrospective, multicenter study of 139 parturients receiving autologous blood transfusion from cell salvage reported no cases of AFE or acute respiratory distress.[80] Maternal alloimmunization is a valid concern given that blood salvage techniques are unable to discriminate between maternal and fetal erythrocytes. Rh antigen discordance is the more significant risk because ABO antigens in the fetus are not well developed. Transfused salvaged blood containing Rh-positive fetal blood could immunize an Rh-negative mother. Thus, after autologous transfusion, the Kleihauer-Betke test is indicated to quantify exposure and calculate the appropriate Rho (D) immune globulin dose to prevent maternal alloimmunization. Provided appropriate precautionary measures are taken to prevent maternal Rh alloimmunization, blood salvage techniques may be especially useful in specific obstetric populations, including rare blood types, Jehovah's Witnesses, and/or limited blood product availability. Several peer-reviewed studies have collectively reported no significant complications to the more than 300 obstetric patients who have received cell-salvaged autologous blood.[75,76,80–84]

SUMMARY

Obstetric hemorrhage remains a significant cause of maternal morbidity and mortality worldwide. Uterine atony, abnormal placentation, genital tract trauma, and coagulation disturbances frequently contribute to massive bleeding in the peripartum period. Given that most obstetric hemorrhage cases occur in the absence of any identifiable risk factor, vigilance is required for the early identification of significant bleeding and hemodynamic instability. Successful management frequently involves stepwise, escalating pharmacologic, hematological, radiological, and/or surgical interventions. It is hoped that universal implementation of obstetric hemorrhage protocols will decrease the frequency of significant adverse outcomes.

REFERENCES

1. Say L, Chou D, Gemmill A, et al. Global causes of maternal death: a WHO systematic analysis. Lancet Glob Health 2014;2(6):e323–33.
2. Cantwell R, Clutton-Brock T, Cooper G, et al. Saving Mothers' Lives: reviewing maternal deaths to make motherhood safer: 2006-2008. The Eighth Report of the Confidential Enquiries into Maternal Deaths in the United Kingdom. BJOG 2011;118(Suppl 1):1–203.
3. Creanga AA, Berg CJ, Syverson C, et al. Pregnancy-related mortality in the united states, 2006-2010. Obstet Gynecol 2015;125(1):5–12.
4. Bateman BT, Berman MF, Riley LE, et al. The epidemiology of postpartum hemorrhage in a large, nationwide sample of deliveries. Anesth Analg 2010;110(5): 1368–73.
5. Abdul-Kadir R, McLintock C, Ducloy AS, et al. Evaluation and management of postpartum hemorrhage: consensus from an international expert panel. Transfusion 2014;54(7):1756–68.
6. Rath WH. Postpartum hemorrhage–update on problems of definitions and diagnosis. Acta Obstet Gynecol Scand 2011;90(5):421–8.
7. Dahlke JD, Mendez-Figueroa H, Maggio L, et al. Prevention and management of postpartum hemorrhage: a comparison of 4 national guidelines. Am J Obstet Gynecol 2015;213(1):76.e1-10.
8. Iyasu S, Saftlas AK, Rowley DL, et al. The epidemiology of placenta previa in the United States, 1979 through 1987. Am J Obstet Gynecol 1993;168(5):1424–9.
9. Cresswell JA, Ronsmans C, Calvert C, et al. Prevalence of placenta praevia by world region: a systematic review and meta-analysis. Trop Med Int Health 2013;18(6):712–24.
10. Silver RM. Abnormal placentation: placenta previa, vasa previa, and placenta accreta. Obstet Gynecol 2015;126(3):654–68.
11. Getahun D, Oyelese Y, Salihu HM, et al. Previous cesarean delivery and risks of placenta previa and placental abruption. Obstet Gynecol 2006;107(4):771–8.
12. Kaczmarczyk M, Sparen P, Terry P, et al. Risk factors for uterine rupture and neonatal consequences of uterine rupture: a population-based study of successive pregnancies in sweden. BJOG 2007;114(10):1208–14.
13. Landon MB, Hauth JC, Leveno KJ, et al. Maternal and perinatal outcomes associated with a trial of labor after prior cesarean delivery. N Engl J Med 2004; 351(25):2581–9.
14. Vedat A, Hasan B, Ismail A. Rupture of the uterus in labor: a review of 150 cases. Isr J Med Sci 1993;29(10):639–43.
15. Alexander JM, Wortman AC. Intrapartum hemorrhage. Obstet Gynecol Clin North Am 2013;40(1):15–26.
16. Salihu HM, Bekan B, Aliyu MH, et al. Perinatal mortality associated with abruptio placenta in singletons and multiples. Am J Obstet Gynecol 2005;193(1):198–203.
17. Tikkanen M, Nuutila M, Hiilesmaa V, et al. Clinical presentation and risk factors of placental abruption. Acta Obstet Gynecol Scand 2006;85(6):700–5.
18. Kramer MS, Berg C, Abenhaim H, et al. Incidence, risk factors, and temporal trends in severe postpartum hemorrhage. Am J Obstet Gynecol 2013;209(5):449.e1-7.
19. Wu S, Kocherginsky M, Hibbard JU. Abnormal placentation: twenty-year analysis. Am J Obstet Gynecol 2005;192(5):1458–61.
20. Comstock CH, Love JJ Jr, Bronsteen RA, et al. Sonographic detection of placenta accreta in the second and third trimesters of pregnancy. Am J Obstet Gynecol 2004;190(4):1135–40.

21. Warshak CR, Eskander R, Hull AD, et al. Accuracy of ultrasonography and magnetic resonance imaging in the diagnosis of placenta accreta. Obstet Gynecol 2006;108(3 Pt 1):573–81.
22. Saleem Z, Rydhstrom H. Vaginal hematoma during parturition: a population-based study. Acta Obstet Gynecol Scand 2004;83(6):560–2.
23. Fahmy K, el-Gazar A, Sammour M, et al. Postpartum colposcopy of the cervix: injury and healing. Int J Gynaecol Obstet 1991;34(2):133–7.
24. Thornton P, Douglas J. Coagulation in pregnancy. Best Pract Res Clin Obstet Gynaecol 2010;24(3):339–52.
25. Girard T, Mortl M, Schlembach D. New approaches to obstetric hemorrhage: the postpartum hemorrhage consensus algorithm. Curr Opin Anaesthesiol 2014;27(3):267–74.
26. Farquhar C, Sadler L, Masson V, et al. Beyond the numbers: classifying contributory factors and potentially avoidable maternal deaths in New Zealand, 2006-2009. Am J Obstet Gynecol 2011;205(4):331.e1-8.
27. Haeri S, Dildy GA 3rd. Maternal mortality from hemorrhage. Semin Perinatol 2012;36(1):48–55.
28. Shields LE, Wiesner S, Fulton J, et al. Comprehensive maternal hemorrhage protocols reduce the use of blood products and improve patient safety. Am J Obstet Gynecol 2015;212(3):272–80.
29. Kacmar RM, Mhyre JM, Scavone BM, et al. The use of postpartum hemorrhage protocols in United States academic obstetric anesthesia units. Anesth Analg 2014;119(4):906–10.
30. Main EK, Goffman D, Scavone BM, et al. National partnership for maternal safety: consensus bundle on obstetric hemorrhage. Anesth Analg 2015;121(1):142–8.
31. Scavone BM, Tung A. The transfusion dilemma: more, less, or more organized? Anesthesiology 2014;121(3):439–41.
32. Bose P, Regan F, Paterson-Brown S. Improving the accuracy of estimated blood loss at obstetric haemorrhage using clinical reconstructions. BJOG 2006;113(8):919–24.
33. Westhoff G, Cotter AM, Tolosa JE. Prophylactic oxytocin for the third stage of labour to prevent postpartum haemorrhage. Cochrane Database Syst Rev 2013;(10):CD001808.
34. Chen M, Chang Q, Duan T, et al. Uterine massage to reduce blood loss after vaginal delivery: a randomized controlled trial. Obstet Gynecol 2013;122(2 Pt 1):290–5.
35. Hofmeyr GJ, Abdel-Aleem H, Abdel-Aleem MA. Uterine massage for preventing postpartum haemorrhage. Cochrane Database Syst Rev 2013;(7):CD006431.
36. Zhao Y, Zhang Y, Li Z. Appropriate second-line therapies for management of severe postpartum hemorrhage. Int J Gynaecol Obstet 2014;127(2):180–2.
37. Kozek-Langenecker SA. Effects of hydroxyethyl starch solutions on hemostasis. Anesthesiology 2005;103(3):654–60.
38. Westphal M, James MF, Kozek-Langenecker S, et al. Hydroxyethyl starches: different products–different effects. Anesthesiology 2009;111(1):187–202.
39. Finfer S, Bellomo R, Boyce N, et al. A comparison of albumin and saline for fluid resuscitation in the intensive care unit. N Engl J Med 2004;350(22):2247–56.
40. Perel P, Roberts I, Ker K. Colloids versus crystalloids for fluid resuscitation in critically ill patients. Cochrane Database Syst Rev 2013;(2):CD000567.
41. Mercier FJ, Bonnet MP. Use of clotting factors and other prohemostatic drugs for obstetric hemorrhage. Curr Opin Anaesthesiol 2010;23(3):310–6.

42. Bolliger D, Szlam F, Molinaro RJ, et al. Finding the optimal concentration range for fibrinogen replacement after severe haemodilution: an in vitro model. Br J Anaesth 2009;102(6):793–9.

43. Santoso JT, Saunders BA, Grosshart K. Massive blood loss and transfusion in obstetrics and gynecology. Obstet Gynecol Surv 2005;60(12):827–37.

44. Ho AM, Dion PW, Cheng CA, et al. A mathematical model for fresh frozen plasma transfusion strategies during major trauma resuscitation with ongoing hemorrhage. Can J Surg 2005;48(6):470–8.

45. Pasquier P, Gayat E, Rackelboom T, et al. An observational study of the fresh frozen plasma: red blood cell ratio in postpartum hemorrhage. Anesth Analg 2013;116(1):155–61.

46. Levy JH, Welsby I, Goodnough LT. Fibrinogen as a therapeutic target for bleeding: a review of critical levels and replacement therapy. Transfusion 2014; 54(5):1389–405 [quiz: 1388].

47. Charbit B, Mandelbrot L, Samain E, et al. The decrease of fibrinogen is an early predictor of the severity of postpartum hemorrhage. J Thromb Haemost 2007; 5(2):266–73.

48. Cortet M, Deneux-Tharaux C, Dupont C, et al. Association between fibrinogen level and severity of postpartum haemorrhage: secondary analysis of a prospective trial. Br J Anaesth 2012;108(6):984–9.

49. de Lloyd L, Bovington R, Kaye A, et al. Standard haemostatic tests following major obstetric haemorrhage. Int J Obstet Anesth 2011;20(2):135–41.

50. Fries D, Martini WZ. Role of fibrinogen in trauma-induced coagulopathy. Br J Anaesth 2010;105(2):116–21.

51. Ahmed S, Harrity C, Johnson S, et al. The efficacy of fibrinogen concentrate compared with cryoprecipitate in major obstetric haemorrhage—an observational study. Transfus Med 2012;22(5):344–9.

52. Bell SF, Rayment R, Collins PW, et al. The use of fibrinogen concentrate to correct hypofibrinogenaemia rapidly during obstetric haemorrhage. Int J Obstet Anesth 2010;19(2):218–23.

53. Kikuchi M, Itakura A, Miki A, et al. Fibrinogen concentrate substitution therapy for obstetric hemorrhage complicated by coagulopathy. J Obstet Gynaecol Res 2013;39(4):770–6.

54. Theusinger OM, Baulig W, Seifert B, et al. Relative concentrations of haemostatic factors and cytokines in solvent/detergent-treated and fresh-frozen plasma. Br J Anaesth 2011;106(4):505–11.

55. Johansson PI, Stensballe J. Effect of haemostatic control resuscitation on mortality in massively bleeding patients: a before and after study. Vox Sang 2009;96(2): 111–8.

56. Nascimento B, Goodnough LT, Levy JH. Cryoprecipitate therapy. Br J Anaesth 2014;113(6):922–34.

57. Theodoulou A, Berryman J, Nathwani A, et al. Comparison of cryoprecipitate with fibrinogen concentrate for acquired hypofibrinogenaemia. Transfus Apher Sci 2012;46(2):159–62.

58. Franchini M. The use of recombinant activated factor VII in platelet disorders: a critical review of the literature. Blood Transfus 2009;7(1):24–8.

59. Hossain N, Shansi T, Haider S, et al. Use of recombinant activated factor VII for massive postpartum hemorrhage. Acta Obstet Gynecol Scand 2007;86(10): 1200–6.

60. Alfirevic Z, Elbourne D, Pavord S, et al. Use of recombinant activated factor VII in primary postpartum hemorrhage: the Northern European Registry 2000-2004. Obstet Gynecol 2007;110(6):1270–8.
61. Phillips LE, McLintock C, Pollock W, et al. Recombinant activated factor VII in obstetric hemorrhage: experiences from the Australian and New Zealand haemostasis registry. Anesth Analg 2009;109(6):1908–15.
62. Yank V, Tuohy CV, Logan AC, et al. Systematic review: benefits and harms of in-hospital use of recombinant factor VIIa for off-label indications. Ann Intern Med 2011;154(8):529–40.
63. Hellgren M. Hemostasis during normal pregnancy and puerperium. Semin Thromb Hemost 2003;29(2):125–30.
64. Henry DA, Carless PA, Moxey AJ, et al. Anti-fibrinolytic use for minimising perioperative allogeneic blood transfusion. Cochrane Database Syst Rev 2011;(3):CD001886.
65. Ker K, Edwards P, Perel P, et al. Effect of tranexamic acid on surgical bleeding: systematic review and cumulative meta-analysis. BMJ 2012;344:e3054.
66. CRASH-2 Trial Collaborators, Shakur H, Roberts I, et al. Effects of tranexamic acid on death, vascular occlusive events, and blood transfusion in trauma patients with significant haemorrhage (CRASH-2): a randomised, placebo-controlled trial. Lancet 2010;376(9734):23–32.
67. Matteson KA, Rahn DD, Wheeler TL 2nd, et al. Nonsurgical management of heavy menstrual bleeding: a systematic review. Obstet Gynecol 2013;121(3): 632–43.
68. Sekhavat L, Tabatabaii A, Dalili M, et al. Efficacy of tranexamic acid in reducing blood loss after cesarean section. J Matern Fetal Neonatal Med 2009;22(1):72–5.
69. Gai MY, Wu LF, Su QF, et al. Clinical observation of blood loss reduced by tranexamic acid during and after caesarian section: a multi-center, randomized trial. Eur J Obstet Gynecol Reprod Biol 2004;112(2):154–7.
70. Gungorduk K, Yildirim G, Asicioglu O, et al. Efficacy of intravenous tranexamic acid in reducing blood loss after elective cesarean section: a prospective, randomized, double-blind, placebo-controlled study. Am J Perinatol 2011;28(3): 233–40.
71. Movafegh A, Eslamian L, Dorabadi A. Effect of intravenous tranexamic acid administration on blood loss during and after cesarean delivery. Int J Gynaecol Obstet 2011;115(3):224–6.
72. Senturk MB, Cakmak Y, Yildiz G, et al. Tranexamic acid for cesarean section: a double-blind, placebo-controlled, randomized clinical trial. Arch Gynecol Obstet 2013;287(4):641–5.
73. Sentilhes L, Lasocki S, Ducloy-Bouthors AS, et al. Tranexamic acid for the prevention and treatment of postpartum haemorrhage. Br J Anaesth 2015;114(4): 576–87.
74. Shakur H, Elbourne D, Gulmezoglu M, et al. The WOMAN trial (World Maternal Antifibrinolytic Trial): tranexamic acid for the treatment of postpartum haemorrhage: an international randomised, double blind placebo controlled trial. Trials 2010;11:40.
75. Goucher H, Wong CA, Patel SK, et al. Cell salvage in obstetrics. Anesth Analg 2015;121(2):465–8.
76. King M, Wrench I, Galimberti A, et al. Introduction of cell salvage to a large obstetric unit: the first six months. Int J Obstet Anesth 2009;18(2):111–7.
77. Waters JH, Tuohy MJ, Hobson DF, et al. Bacterial reduction by cell salvage washing and leukocyte depletion filtration. Anesthesiology 2003;99(3):652–5.

78. Waters JH, Biscotti C, Potter PS, et al. Amniotic fluid removal during cell salvage in the cesarean section patient. Anesthesiology 2000;92(6):1531–6.
79. Catling SJ, Williams S, Fielding AM. Cell salvage in obstetrics: an evaluation of the ability of cell salvage combined with leucocyte depletion filtration to remove amniotic fluid from operative blood loss at caesarean section. Int J Obstet Anesth 1999;8(2):79–84.
80. Rebarber A, Lonser R, Jackson S, et al. The safety of intraoperative autologous blood collection and autotransfusion during cesarean section. Am J Obstet Gynecol 1998;179(3 Pt 1):715–20.
81. Tevet A, Grisaru-Granovsky S, Samueloff A, et al. Peripartum use of cell salvage: a university practice audit and literature review. Arch Gynecol Obstet 2012; 285(2):281–4.
82. Rainaldi MP, Tazzari PL, Scagliarini G, et al. Blood salvage during caesarean section. Br J Anaesth 1998;80(2):195–8.
83. Elagamy A, Abdelaziz A, Ellaithy M. The use of cell salvage in women undergoing cesarean hysterectomy for abnormal placentation. Int J Obstet Anesth 2013; 22(4):289–93.
84. Pahlavan P, Nezhat C, Nezhat C. Hemorrhage in obstetrics and gynecology. Curr Opin Obstet Gynecol 2001;13(4):419–24.

The Use of Ultrasonography in Obstetric Anesthesia

Chiraag Talati, MBBS, BSc (Hons), FRCA[a], Cristian Arzola, MD, MSc[b],
Jose C.A. Carvalho, MD, PhD, FANZCA, FRCPC[c,d],*

KEYWORDS

- Ultrasound • Ultrasonography • Anesthesia • Obstetric

KEY POINTS

- Some national guidelines advocate the placement of central vascular access with ultrasonography when possible, and this applies to the obstetric cohort, who may otherwise be technically difficult because of body habitus and edema.
- Pre-procedural spinal ultrasonography assessment facilitates the placement of neuraxial anesthesia, and national guidelines for ultrasonography-assisted epidural catheter placement have been issued. It reduces the number of attempts, ensures a higher success rate, and is helpful for predicted difficult insertions, such as in obese individuals and those with scoliosis.
- Many clinical situations in obstetrics call for urgent interventions, when fasting status is unclear. Gastric ultrasound provides a qualitative and quantitative assessment of the gastric content, and may be useful in estimating perioperative aspiration risk.
- Lung ultrasound is a novel concept in the obstetric population, but it is well-established in the critical care setting. It is particularly useful in diagnosing pulmonary edema, and the consequent progression or resolution of the disease process. Its role in severe preeclampsia and heart failure may be advantageous, especially without the concerns of ionizing radiation that are present in current imaging tools.

Continued

Disclosure: The authors have no financial or nonfinancial relationships to disclose.
[a] Department of Anaesthesia, Homerton University Hospital NHS Foundation Trust, Homerton Row, London E9 6SR, UK; [b] Department of Anesthesia and Pain Management, Mount Sinai Hospital, University of Toronto, 600 University Avenue, Room 19-104, Toronto, Ontario M5G 1X5, Canada; [c] Department of Anesthesia and Pain Management, Mount Sinai Hospital, University of Toronto, 600 University Avenue, Room 19-103, Toronto, Ontario M5G 1X5, Canada; [d] Department of Obstetrics and Gynecology, Mount Sinai Hospital, University of Toronto, 600 University Avenue, Room 19-103, Toronto, Ontario M5G 1X5, Canada
* Corresponding author. Mount Sinai Hospital, 600 University Avenue, Room 19-103, Toronto, Ontario M5G 1X5, Canada.
E-mail address: jose.carvalho@uhn.ca

Anesthesiology Clin 35 (2017) 35–58
http://dx.doi.org/10.1016/j.anclin.2016.09.005
1932-2275/17/© 2016 Elsevier Inc. All rights reserved.

Continued

- Postoperative analgesia can be improved by transversus abdominis plane blocks. Direct real-time ultrasonography guidance of the needle adds an extra level of safety to this procedure.
- Accurate identification of the cricothyroid membrane is a key skill for anesthesiologists, and is typically performed poorly by palpation. Ultrasonography can aid precise localization of the cricothyroid membrane for successful, life-saving cricothyrotomy.

INTRODUCTION

In recent years, advancements in technology have revolutionized the practice of anesthesia. In particular, the different applications of ultrasonography in anesthesia have made significant progress, proving ultrasonography to be an indispensable tool. Some national guidelines have recommended that procedures such as central venous access and peripheral nerve blocks be performed under ultrasonography as a standard among anesthesiologists.[1-3]

For decades, obstetric clinicians have used ultrasonography for the assessment and management of fetal and maternal well-being; consequently the labor suite is well acquainted with its application. The portability, cost-effectiveness, and nonionizing nature of this imaging modality lends itself as a central resource in obstetrics. Therefore, applying ultrasonography in obstetric anesthesia is a natural way forward.

The incidence of complex medical problems among the obstetric population is increasing,[4] and anesthesia for parturients is prone to such complexities. Ultrasonography provides accurate visualization of internal anatomic structures that can facilitate assessment of clinical conditions and increase the safety of therapeutic interventions.

Assessment purposes include evaluation of gastric content to help estimate the risk of pulmonary aspiration, as well as the investigation of dyspnea using lung ultrasonography. From a safety perspective, the cricothyroid membrane can be identified and preemptively marked in anticipated difficult airway cases. Therapeutic interventions such as neuraxial anesthesia, transversus abdominis plane (TAP) block, and vascular access can be performed effectively and with a reduction of risk when performed under ultrasonography guidance.

This article describes the indications, techniques, and future directions of ultrasonography in obstetric anesthesia, and focuses on its use for neuraxial anesthesia, TAP block, cricothyroid membrane identification, vascular access, gastric content assessment, and lung disorder diagnosis.

ULTRASOUND PROBES AND PLANES

For the use of ultrasound in obstetric anesthesia as described in this chapter, two probes are used: the linear high-frequency probe and the curved low-frequency probe. **Table 1** shows the key features of each probe.

Two main planes of the probe are described in this article (**Fig. 1**):

- Longitudinal, which refers to positioning the probe in a vertical axis. This can be:
  - Midline
  - Paramedian
- Transverse, which refers to holding the probe in a horizontal axis.

Table 1
Characteristics and uses of linear and curved ultrasound probes

	Linear Probe	Curved Probe
Frequency	High 15–7 MHz	Low 5–2 MHz
Depth penetration	Superficial	Deep
Field of view	Narrow	Wide
Resolution	Higher	Lower
Uses	Vascular TAP block Cricothyroid membrane Lung	Spinal Gastric Lung

KEY AREAS FOR THE USE OF ULTRASONOGRAPHY IN OBSTETRIC ANESTHESIA
Neuraxial Anesthesia Placement

Nature of the problem
Effective and safe neuraxial blockade is a fundamental aspect of obstetric anesthesia. The placement of spinal or epidural anesthesia is traditionally based on the palpation of surface landmarks. In several circumstances, such as obesity, edema, and scoliosis, these landmarks can be difficult to identify. Even when surface landmarks are successfully identified, anesthesiologists may fail to acknowledge the desired interspace. MRI has shown that anesthesiologists are correct in less than 30% of identifications of interspaces by the palpatory technique, and the error can be as much as 4 interspaces. In almost all of the errors, clinicians are higher than assumed, and, for intrathecal injection, this has significant safety implications.[5]

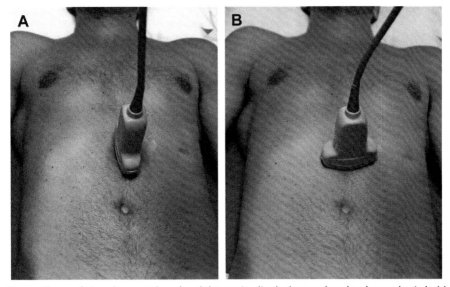

Fig. 1. Plane of the ultrasound probe. (*A*) Longitudinal plane, whereby the probe is held vertically, which can be midline or paramedian. (*B*) Transverse plane, whereby the probe is held horizontally.

Spinal ultrasonography has gained significant popularity in the past decade. Equipped with the information provided by preprocedural ultrasonography, novice trainees have shown a significant higher success rate of epidural placement.[6] This finding has also been confirmed by a recent meta-analysis reviewing epidural catheter placement or lumbar puncture with the aid of ultrasonography, which found fewer:

- Failed attempts
- Needle redirections
- Traumatic attempts[7]

Indications for spinal ultrasonography

In the United Kingdom, national guidelines have been issued regarding the facilitation of epidural space catheterization with the use of spinal ultrasonography.[8] Preprocedural spinal ultrasonography can provide a plethora of information for clinicians. It can assist in the identification of the:

- Desired interspace
- Optimal puncture site
- Angle of needle insertion and trajectory
- Estimated depth to the epidural space

Particularly in cases of obesity and scoliosis, neuraxial anesthesia can be challenging. In both patient populations, ultrasound facilitation resulted in only half the number of insertion attempts and needle passes, in addition to a twice as high first-attempt success rate, when compared with the landmark technique.[9] Furthermore, it guides the operator in selecting the appropriate needle length from the outset, by predicting the depth of the epidural space, especially in obese parturients.

Technique

Preprocedural spinal ultrasonography can be performed with the patient in the sitting position. The aim is to identify and mark the optimal puncture site, recognise the angle of needle insertion and estimate the depth to the epidural space. Insertion of neuraxial anesthesia can then proceed as per the anesthesiologist's usual technique.

Spinal sonoanatomy is assessed using a low-frequency curved ultrasound probe, which permits deeper penetration of the ultrasonography beam, increasing the visualization of the structures at the appropriate depth. Valuable information is obtained via 2 viewing approaches: the longitudinal paramedian approach and the transverse midline approach.

Longitudinal paramedian approach Parallel to the long axis of the spine, the probe is held vertically over the sacral area. It is initially placed 2 to 3 cm to the left or to the right of the midline, and angled slightly medially to focus on the center of the spinal canal (**Fig. 2**A). A continuous hyperechoic (bright) line is visualized, which is consistent with the sacrum. As the probe is advanced in a cephalad direction, a hyperechoic sawlike image is observed (**Fig. 2**B). The teeth of the saw correspond to the laminae of each vertebra, and the gaps between the teeth represent the intervertebral spaces. Therefore, advancing the probe in a cephalad direction, clinicians can determine the exact desired interspace on the skin. At each intervertebral space (**Fig. 2**C), 3 important structures are identified, from superficial to deep (**Fig. 2**D):

- Posterior unit: Ligamentum flavum and posterior dura mater
- Intrathecal space
- Anterior unit: anterior dura mater, posterior longitudinal ligament, and vertebral body[10]

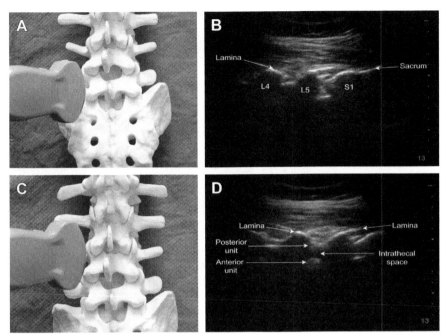

Fig. 2. Longitudinal paramedian approach. (*A*) Ultrasound probe over the sacrum and lower lumbar spine. (*B*) Corresponding sonogram to *A*: hyperechoic image of the sacrum and of the saw sign, the teeth of which represent the laminae of the lumbar vertebrae, and the gaps represent the interspaces. (*C*) Ultrasound probe more cephalad on the lumbar spine. (*D*) Corresponding sonogram to *C*: laminae of 2 adjacent vertebrae and elements of an interspace; from superficial to deep, there is visualization of the posterior unit, the intrathecal space, and the anterior unit. Posterior unit, ligamentum flavum and posterior dura mater; anterior unit, anterior dura mater, posterior longitudinal ligament, and vertebral body.

Transverse midline approach Having located the desired interspaces with the longitudinal approach, more information can be captured with transverse scanning of an interspace. The probe should be held horizontally at the marked level, and perpendicular to the long axis of the spine (**Fig. 3**A). The following actions, in order, can then be undertaken:

- Identify the midline of the spine by visualizing the tip of the spinous process, which is represented by a small hyperechoic signal immediately under the skin. This signal continues as a long triangular hypoechoic image (dark shadow) (**Fig. 3**B).
- Move the probe slightly caudad or cephalad to obtain a good view of the desired interspace (**Fig. 3**C). A good view shows a flying-bat pattern that represents (**Fig. 3**D):
  - The posterior unit
  - Intrathecal space
  - Anterior unit
  - Paramedian structures such as the articular and transverse processes
- At this point, freeze the image.
- The probe should be held steady, and 2 points are marked on the skin:
  - Midline point: matching with the center of the upper horizontal surface of the probe

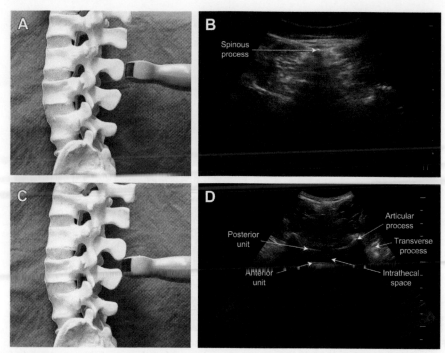

Fig. 3. Transverse midline approach. (*A*) Ultrasound probe at the tip of a lumbar spinous process. (*B*) Corresponding sonogram to *A*: the tip of the spinous process appears as a small hyperechoic structure immediately beneath the skin, and determines a long vertical black hypoechoic shadow. (*C*) Ultrasound probe at a lumbar interspace. (*D*) Corresponding sonogram to *C*: typical interspace showing the flying-bat sign. Within the interspace, from superficial to deep, there is visualization of the posterior unit, the intrathecal space, and the anterior unit. Paramedian structures such as the articular and transverse processes can also be visualized. Posterior unit, ligamentum flavum and posterior dura mater; anterior unit, anterior dura mater, posterior longitudinal ligament, and vertebral body.

- ○ Interspace point: matching with the middle point of the right lateral surface of the probe
- At the intersection of these 2 points, the puncture site is determined (**Fig. 4**).
- On the frozen image, the depth to the epidural space can be accurately measured:
  - ○ Identify the posterior unit, which is formed by the ligamentum flavum and posterior dura mater
  - ○ Use built-in calipers on the screen to measure the distance from the skin to the inner side of the posterior unit
  - ○ When capturing the frozen image, try to keep the degree of compression of the subcutaneous tissue by the probe to a minimum, because underestimation of the depth to the epidural space may occur with any degree of compression[10]

Successful puncture Although the optimal puncture site has been determined, the angle of needle insertion and needle trajectory are key. The angle of needle insertion should reproduce the angle at which the ultrasound probe was held to obtain the best image of the flying bat.

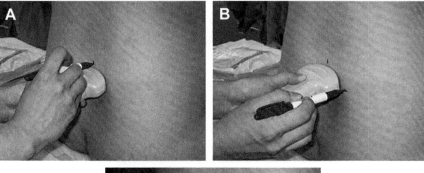

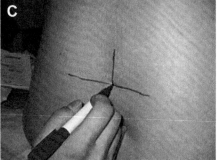

Fig. 4. Determination of the puncture point. On visualizing a clear image of the interspace, the image is frozen and the probe held steady. (*A*) A point at the center of the upper horizontal surface is marked. (*B*) A point at the middle point of the right lateral surface of the probe is marked. (*C*) At the intersection of the extensions of these 2 points, the puncture site is determined. (*From* Carvalho JCA. Ultrasound-facilitated epidural and spinals in obstetrics. Anesthesiol Clin 2008;26(1):153; with permission.)

Assessment of Gastric Content

Nature of the problem

Pulmonary aspiration of gastric contents under general anesthesia is a serious complication for anesthesiologists. It carries a significant risk of morbidity and mortality, first described by Curtis Mendelson[11] in 1946. He acknowledged 3 major determinants of the risk of morbidity and mortality:

- Gastric pH
- Gastric volume
- Gastric content: solid food boluses could result in asphyxiation

Particularly in obstetric anesthesia, in which urgent operative interventions are required in patients with questionable fasting status, an insight into the gastric volume and content is advantageous, and has the ability to influence clinical decision making.

Gastric ultrasonography has recently gained popularity among anesthesiologists as a potential tool to estimate the risk of aspiration at the bedside. Gastric ultrasonography can provide both qualitative and quantitative information relating to the nature and volume of the gastric content respectively.[12] However, clinicians must understand that gastric volume and contents are surrogate end points only, and are only indirect measurements of aspiration risk.[13]

Although gastric ultrasonography is currently not used in routine practice, it has made great progress in the past decade as a research tool. It has shown that:

- Gastric emptying times are similar in third-trimester nonlaboring pregnant women and in nonpregnant women.[14]
- Ingestion of moderate amounts of clear fluid does not delay gastric emptying in third-trimester nonlaboring women.[15]
- There is no difference in clear fluid gastric emptying of obese compared with nonobese nonlaboring women at term.[16]
- Previous studies have suggested delayed gastric emptying during labor via ultrasonography, with the frequent finding of solid contents despite a fast of 8 to 24 hours.[17] However, recent evidence has shown that women in labor under epidural analgesia and kept fasted show a reduction in their antral size as per serial gastric ultrasonography, indicating preserved gastric motility.[18]
- Isotonic drinks consumed during labor are rapidly emptied from the stomach.[19]

Although the existing literature on gastric ultrasonography assessment has reinforced current fasting guidelines in nonlaboring pregnant women, it has also suggested that labor provides a variable response to gastric emptying. Therefore, bedside ultrasonography may provide a safe, prompt, and effective means of assessment of the risk of pulmonary aspiration in laboring parturients.

Indications for gastric ultrasonography
Bedside ultrasonography still requires investigation before it can be used as a clinical tool for aspiration risk estimation, and its implications for clinical care remain unknown. However, gastric ultrasonography assessment could be clinically indicated in several instances:

- When the fasting status is unknown, because of issues surrounding communication barriers or patient understanding.
- In a nonelective setting, when clinicians would otherwise delay a procedure for insufficient timing of fasting and proceed after the fasting guidelines have been met.
- When a patient has met the fasting guidelines but clinical suspicion of delayed gastric emptying is high; for example, administration of parental or enteral opioids.

Technique
Visualization of the whole stomach can be challenging. The presence of air can make the body of the stomach in particular difficult to view. The fundus is generally a deep structure that may also contain air and therefore can be difficult to visualize.[12,20] Hence, the antrum is the optimal part of the stomach to scan for the following reasons:

- It is the most amenable and easily accessible part of the stomach
- It contains the smallest volume of air
- It maintains a consistent, identifiable shape
- It is thought that its assessment accurately represents the findings of the rest of the stomach[20]

In order to optimize the views of the antrum, the patient should be in a 45° semirecumbent right lateral decubitus position; this helps air rise proximally toward the fundus, and fluid/semifluid content gravitate toward the antrum, for an accurate assessment.[20]

Given the depth of the antrum, a low-frequency curved probe is best suited for gastric scanning. The probe is held in a longitudinal plane (**Fig. 5**), placed at the left subcostal margin, and moved in a fanlike manner from the left toward the right

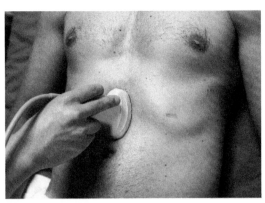

Fig. 5. Probe positioning in gastric ultrasonography. The probe is held longitudinally beginning in the left subcostal margin and is moved toward the midline and the right subcostal area.

subcostal area, over the epigastric region. The antrum can be visualized between the left lobe of the liver (anteriorly) and the body of the pancreas (posteriorly), usually just right of the abdominal midline. Particularly useful landmarks include the inferior vena cava and aorta. The probe can be turned clockwise or counterclockwise to improve the antral view.[12]

The antrum can be assessed for the qualitative nature of gastric content: empty, clear fluid, or solid food. **Fig. 6** shows the ultrasonographic appearances of the various fasting states, and **Table 2** summarizes a description of the findings.

Similarly, the quantitative nature of gastric volume can be calculated in the longitudinal plane of the antrum scan. Several formulas exist, based on the cross-sectional area of the antrum, but until now they have been developed for nonpregnant adults positioned in the right lateral decubitus and only for clear fluid content.[20]

Assessment of Dyspnea

Nature of the problem
Lung ultrasonography is a fairly novel concept in obstetrics; however, it has been used in routine practice for diagnosis and therapeutic intervention in intensive care medicine for several years. There is a lack of data for the use and feasibility of lung ultrasonography in the obstetric population. Ultrasonography of the chest in this patient population is a reasonable alternative to the traditional imaging modalities, such as chest radiographs and computed tomography, which are relatively contraindicated in pregnancy.

Pregnant women in the third trimester have significantly altered lung physiology and respiratory parameters. Dyspnea is common in this patient population, and differentiating disorder from normal physiology of pregnancy can be problematic. The availability of a noninvasive, safe, and accurate tool for pulmonary assessment in routine clinical practice is essential. Pulmonary edema is common, and can complicate up to 0.5% of pregnancies. Identification of patients at risk of pulmonary edema is therefore a topic of interest.[21]

Indications for lung ultrasonography
Ultrasonography of the lung is an important tool in the initial assessment of dyspnea. It could direct therapeutic interventions or guide further investigations.

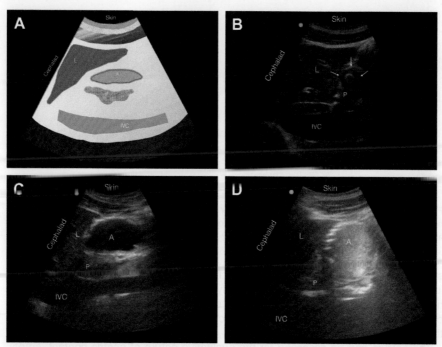

Fig. 6. Gastric ultrasonography and the appearance of the antrum. (A) Schematic illustration of the antrum. (B) Empty antrum showing bull's-eye target. (C) 200 mL of clear fluid showing starry-night appearance. (D) Recent ingestion of solid food contents shown by a frosted glass appearance and difficult visualization due to air. Arrows show the bull's eye target. A, antrum; IVC, inferior vena cava; L, liver; P, pancreas.

Table 2		
Description of the antrum seen on gastric ultrasonography in an empty state, and following clear fluid and a solid meal		
Empty	**Clear Fluid (200 mL)**	**Solid Meal**
• Collapsed, flat	• Distended	At 5 min:
• Thick walls	• Round	• A frosted glass appearance, which is hyperechoic
• Anterior and posterior walls close together, and round/oval: bull's eye target appearance	• Thin gastric walls	• Air-solid mixture creates ring-down artifacts.
	• Hypoechoic fluid content	• This impairs visualization of deeper structures
	• When seen immediately after ingestion: starry-night appearance	At 90 min:
		• More homogeneous character, after air is displaced
		• Intermediate echogenicity
		• Allows deeper structures to be visualized

Data from Cubillos J, Tse C, Chan VW, et al. Bedside ultrasound assessment of gastric content: an observational study. Can J Anaesth 2012;59(4):416–23.

An international consensus of experts concluded that the diagnoses of pulmonary edema, pneumothorax, and lung consolidation are either more accurate or of equal accuracy by lung ultrasonography compared with chest radiographs.[22] As a skill, one study showed that physicians can readily recognize key artifacts leading to the diagnosis of pulmonary edema and pneumothorax following training with a brief learning module in thoracic ultrasonography.[23]

One particular advantage of lung ultrasonography in the obstetric population is the ability to monitor progression or resolution of respiratory disorders through the course of disease, as a safe and cost-effective modality. Specifically, it can monitor lung reaeration in disease states such as pulmonary edema, acute lung injury, and pneumonia.[22] Serial scanning can be undertaken to monitor the response to therapy, and tailor treatment accordingly. Ultrasonography of the lung seems particularly useful for monitoring pulmonary edema. Before alveolar edema develops, there is a silent phase of interstitial edema, which can be easily detected on ultrasonography. Therefore, lung ultrasonography can be used in patient groups at risk for developing pulmonary edema, such as preeclampsia, and be used as a risk reduction tool.[24] It could also be used to prevent harmful fluid intake in patients found to be at risk.

Technique
For a thorough examination of the anterior chest, a detailed approach can be undertaken by the 28-rib space technique. To undertake this examination (**Fig. 7**):

- Each hemithorax is divided into 4 segments:
  - Upper anterior
  - Lower anterior
  - Upper lateral
  - Basal lateral
- On the left hemithorax:
  - The second, third, and fourth rib spaces are assessed, totaling 12 views
- On the right hemithorax:
  - The second, third, fourth, and fifth rib spaces are assessed, totaling 16 views[24]

With the patient in the supine position, a curved low-frequency or linear high-frequency probe is applied in a longitudinal plane and is held vertically and perpendicular to the ribs (**Fig. 8**A). On application of the probe, the clinician immediately sees (**Fig. 8**B):

- Superior and inferior rib posterior shadows appearing as horizontal hyperechoic lines.
- Deeper to this, and between the center of these shadows, another horizontal hyperechoic sliding line is visible, which is the pleural line (lung sliding).
- Deep to the pleural line, horizontal artifacts can normally be seen. These are called A-lines.
- Lung pulse: the subtle rhythmic movement of visceral on parietal pleura with cardiac oscillations.[22,24]

A wide range of disorders can be detected on lung ultrasonography.

Interstitial edema This mainly refers to pulmonary edema, but it can include interstitial pneumonia or diffuse parenchymal lung disease. Interstitial edema is typically shown by the presence of reverberation artifacts called B-lines, which are produced by the increased density of lung tissue (**Fig. 9**). They appear as discrete, vertical, hyperechoic lines initiating from the pleural line, extending to the bottom of the screen without fading, and moving synchronously with lung sliding.[22,24]

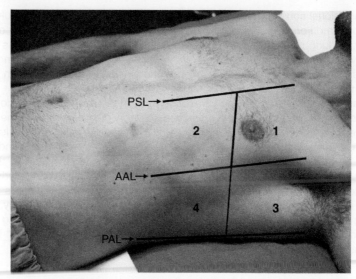

Fig. 7. Twenty-eight-rib space technique allows a detailed examination of the chest. The left hemithorax is divided into 4 segments: the upper (1) and lower (2) anterior chest, and the upper (3) and basal (4) lateral chest. The right hemithorax is divided into 4 similar segments. On the right and left hemithorax, 16 and 12 views are obtained respectively. AAL, anterior axillary line; PAL, posterior axillary line; PSL, parasternal line.

A B-pattern is the presence of 3 or more B-lines on each side of the anterior chest, and this satisfies a diagnosis of pulmonary edema. In the critical care setting, this has a sensitivity of 100% and specificity of 92% for diagnosing pulmonary edema.[22–24] In addition, the number of B-lines can help indicate the severity of congestion.[22] The presence of focal multiple B-lines may be seen in pneumonia, atelectasis, pulmonary infarction, pleural disease, and malignancy.[22]

Pneumothorax The diagnosis of pneumothorax on lung ultrasonography is a basic technique with the following characteristics:

- Absence of lung sliding
- Absence of B-lines

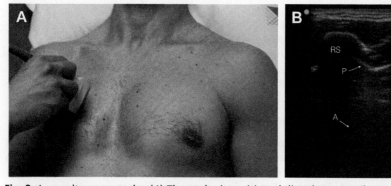

Fig. 8. Lung ultrasonography. (A) The probe is positioned directly over a rib space. (B) Corresponding sonoanatomy of a normal rib space, with superior and inferior rib shadows, pleura, and A-lines. A, A-line; P, pleura; RI, inferior rib; RS, superior rib.

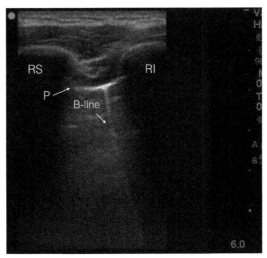

Fig. 9. Lung ultrasonography showing a B-line, which is seen with increased density of lung tissue. Multiple B-lines are termed a B-pattern appearance, satisfying the diagnosis of pulmonary edema. B, B-line; P, pleura; RI, inferior rib; RS, superior rib.

- Absence of lung pulse
- Presence of lung points: the transition point of an absence of lung sliding to the presence of lung sliding indicates the limit of the pneumothorax[22]

Lung consolidation Lung consolidation can also be diagnosed with accuracy on ultrasonography, and images show an echo-poor or tissuelike image, depending on the extent of air loss and predominance of fluid.[22]

Pleural effusion In all free pleural effusions, both of the following signs are present:

- Anechoic space between parietal and visceral pleura
- Sinusoid sign: respiratory movement of the lung within the effusion, better visualized on M-mode[22]

Postoperative Analgesia

Nature of the problem
Neural block of the somatic afferent input of the abdominal wall is an effective mode of postoperative analgesia in patients undergoing cesarean delivery. This block can be achieved by bilateral TAP blocks, and recently this technique has gained popularity, especially under real-time ultrasonographic guidance.

The anterolateral abdominal wall has an afferent neural supply from the anterior rami of spinal nerves T7 to L1, including the ilioinguinal and iliohypogastric nerves. These nerves run in a continuous fascial plane, known as the TAP, between the internal oblique and transversus abdominis muscles. Deposition of local anesthetic at a single point in this space permits spread along this plane and effective analgesia for up to 36 hours.[25]

The TAP is awkwardly close to the peritoneum and the potential for inadvertent visceral injury is real. In the past, the block was undertaken with a blind or landmark technique, which relied on a popping sensation following piercing of fascial planes with a blunt needle. This end point is subjective, and can be unreliable. When anesthesiologists who regularly performed this landmark technique were assessed, an expert ultrasonographer examined the position of their needle tips. The needle was in the correct position in less than 24% of the attempts. Of concern, the needle was intraperitoneal in 18% of cases and was in a layer of muscle in approximately 50% of cases. The study was rightfully terminated early because of the identification of highly unacceptable wrong placement rates.[26] The literature describes cases of colonic perforation and liver puncture with blind abdominal plane blocks.[27] Using real-time ultrasonography to facilitate TAP blocks ensures a higher safety profile.[28]

Indications for ultrasonography-guided TAP block

TAP block is preferred for lower abdominal surgery, below the level of the umbilicus, because local anesthetic spread above T10 is rare. Therefore, it lends itself particularly well as a postoperative analgesia adjunct for lower segment cesarean delivery.

The use of TAP blocks could be considered for cesarean delivery in urgent cases or for patients with a contraindication to neuraxial block. In these patients undergoing general anesthesia, TAP blocks can be a useful tool for multimodal analgesia. In addition, a particular advantage of TAP blocks is the preservation of hemodynamic stability, compared with neuraxial anesthesia.

Although it cannot be used as an alternative to neuraxial anesthesia, it can be combined with neuraxial blockade. When TAP blocks are performed in conjunction with spinal anesthesia without long-acting intrathecal opioids, investigations have shown significantly reduced morphine requirements, reduced antiemetic use, far superior analgesia at 48 hours, and improved patient satisfaction.[25,29] One meta-analysis found that TAP blocks were an effective analgesic option when neuraxial morphine was not used.[30] Therefore TAP blocks could be considered as an adjunct to spinal or epidural anesthesia when neuraxial or systemic long-acting opioids are undesirable in specific patients (eg, sensitivity to morphine, or obstructive sleep apnea).

Technique

TAP blocks are performed using a high-frequency linear probe. The patient should be supine, with arms abducted for direct access to the abdominal wall. Because the block is performed with real-time ultrasonography guidance, prepare the ultrasound probe and abdominal wall for an aseptic technique.

Begin ultrasonography scanning in a transverse plane, at the midpoint between the iliac crest and costal margin, in line with the midaxillary line (**Fig. 10**). To improve the view, the probe can be glided onto more anterior abdominal wall. This position may help identify the abdominal wall muscles. The probe can then be glided back laterally, and the muscle layers followed. The final position of the probe must not be more anterior than the anterior axillary line.

Once the probe is in a good position, and the muscles (from superficial to deep: external oblique, internal oblique, and transversus abdominis) and TAP identified (**Fig. 11**), the block can be performed.

The authors advise that the block be performed with an in-plane technique, which permits visualization of the needle shaft and tip throughout the procedure. A 22-G 100-mm block needle is used, and the direction of needle insertion is always medial to lateral (**Fig. 12**). The needle is introduced 2 cm medial to the probe. The probe can then be positioned near the needle entry point to follow the needle in its early superficial path. As the needle ascends forward and deeper, the probe can slowly be returned to its original position. As the needle tip reaches the TAP, 1 to 2 mL of normal saline can be injected slowly to confirm correct needle placement and expansion of the plane, which appear as an increasing hypoechoic space. This stage can be followed by injection of the local anesthetic, preceded by aspiration to prevent intravascular injection.

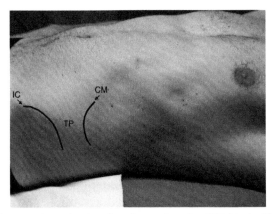

Fig. 10. The surface anatomy landmarks of scanning for TAP block. The probe position should be transverse, and at the midpoint of the costal margin and iliac crest, in the midaxillary line. CM, costal margin; IC, iliac crest; TP, transducer probe.

Note that, for surgical incisions crossing the midline (eg, cesarean delivery), bilateral TAP blocks need to be performed.

Central Vascular Access

Nature of the problem

One of the major uses of ultrasonography by anesthesiologists has been for facilitation of vascular catheterization, which includes central and peripheral venous access, as well as arterial access. Catheterization of central veins has risks, which include arterial puncture; multiple attempts; severe bruising and hematoma; nerve injury; and local structure damage, including pneumothorax and hemothorax.

In some countries, national guidelines recommend the use of ultrasonography for central venous access, specifically internal jugular and femoral vein cannulation.[1,2] The indications for performing subclavian vein catheterization under ultrasonography guidance are equivocal, given the technical difficulties and poor visualization secondary to the bony surroundings.

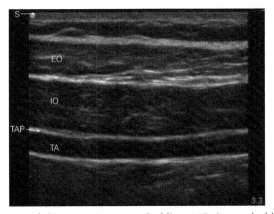

Fig. 11. Sonoanatomy of the TAP. EO, external oblique; IO, internal oblique; S, skin; TA, transversus abdominis.

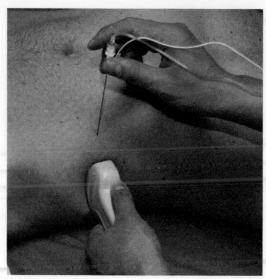

Fig. 12. Needle technique for TAP block. An in-plane technique, showing the needle moving from a medial to lateral direction.

Ultrasonography is ideally performed in real time, but a quick scan can also be undertaken preprocedure to review the anatomy, highlight any technical difficulties from the onset, and select an alternative site if indicated. Most anesthesiologists use ultrasonography routinely in all central vein cannulations. Some may reserve it for predicted difficult cases, such as patients with short neck, obesity, or local scarring caused by radiation therapy. Ultrasonography provides an insight into the anatomy of the vessel and the surrounding structures. It allows clinicians to:

- Select a vein or portion of a vein with a good caliber
- Select a vein or portion of a vein not intimately related to an artery
- Detect thrombosis within a vein and select an alternative site, thereby avoiding the potential associated pitfalls

Compared directly with the landmark technique, internal jugular or femoral vein catheterization with ultrasonography shows a reduction in:

- Failed catheter placements
- Failure on first attempt
- Catheter-related complications (including severe bruising, arterial puncture)
- Attempts to achieve successful catheterization
- Time taken for successful cannulation[1,31]

Indications for ultrasonography-guided vascular access
The indications for using ultrasonography to facilitate vascular access are directed at improving success and minimizing complications in the obstetric population.

Patients in the third trimester have marked physiologic changes of pregnancy. If central venous access is indicated in these patients, clinicians may wish to minimize the risk of inadvertent complications that could be catastrophic. For example, ultrasonography-guided insertion of an internal jugular vein catheter may reduce the chances of a hemothorax or pneumothorax in a parturient with a preexisting decrease in functional residual capacity; or carotid artery puncture causing a hematoma and airway compression in the setting of a preexisting edematous and difficult airway.

Patients with severe preeclampsia often warrant invasive arterial monitoring, and, because of severe edema and vasoconstriction, this can be challenging. Ultrasonography could be used to facilitate this process. It could also be used to help peripheral intravenous access in challenging patient groups by identifying deep veins in the forearm for successful puncture.

Technique

To perform central venous access, the selected sites preferably amenable to ultrasonographic guidance are the internal jugular vein and the femoral vein. In undertaking these procedures, the positioning and preparation of the patient should be as for a landmark technique: supine with a degree of Trendelenburg and the head turned in the opposite direction for internal jugular vein access; and supine with slight abduction of the ipsilateral lower limb for femoral vein access. Utmost care must be taken for aseptic precautions in preparation of the ultrasound probe with sterile gel and a sterile sheath, to minimize the risk of microbial infection of indwelling central catheters.

A high-frequency linear ultrasound probe is used to facilitate vascular access because the structures are of a shallow depth. To identify the internal jugular vein, the ultrasound probe is placed in a transverse plane on the anterior triangle of the neck, which is bordered:

- Anteriorly by the midline
- Posteriorly by the anterior border of the sternocleidomastoid
- Superiorly by the base of the triangle, the mandible

The probe can be glided caudad or cephalad for optimal views. Typically, the internal jugular vein is easily visualized lying superolateral to the carotid artery (**Fig. 13**A). To identify the femoral vein, the probe is positioned in a transverse plane just below the base of the femoral triangle: the superior border of the inguinal ligament. The femoral vein is usually identified medial to the femoral artery (**Fig. 13**B).

Table 3 shows typical ultrasonographic features that can help distinguish arteries from veins.

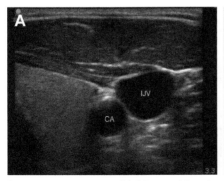
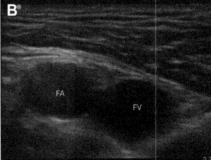

Fig. 13. Sonoanatomy of (A) internal jugular vein and (B) femoral vein. CA, carotid artery; FA, femoral artery; FV, femoral vein; IJV, internal jugular vein.

Table 3
Ultrasonographic features that can help differentiate an artery from a vein

	Artery	Vein
Shape	Round	Oval
Size	Typically smaller	Typically larger
Pulsatile	Yes	No
		Vein changes with respiration
Compressibility (on downward pressure of the probe)	Remains open	Collapses (except if thrombus present)
Valsalva	No effect	Distends internal jugular vein
Color Doppler flow	Toward probe is blue, away from probe is red	

Once the desired vein has been identified, the operator can decide to use an in-plane or an out-of-plane approach to puncture the vein under ultrasonography guidance:

- Out-of-plane approach (short-axis view):
  - ○ This requires the probe to be in a transverse plane and therefore provides a cross-sectional view of the vein (**Fig. 14**A).
  - ○ This approach has a much shorter learning curve.
  - ○ However, it can lead to errors in depth perception, because it cannot provide a view of the whole needle shaft.
  - ○ To view the tip throughout the skin to vein puncture, the probe needs to move either in a cephalad (for femoral vein) or caudad (for internal jugular vein) direction as the needle progresses forward.
- In-plane approach (long-axis view):
  - ○ This requires the probe to be in a longitudinal plane and therefore provides a view of the length of the vein (**Fig. 14**B).
  - ○ The artery cannot be seen in the image, unless it lies directly under the vein.
  - ○ This approach provides a view of the entire needle path, and it can prevent the tip of the needle from penetrating the posterior vein wall.

Investigators have recently shown that an approach in between the long-axis view and short-axis view, also known as the oblique-axis approach, uses strengths of each technique. It allows imaging of surrounding structures, as well as permitting needle

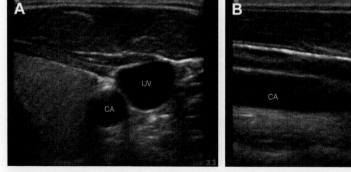

Fig. 14. Sonoanatomy of internal jugular vein. (*A*) Out-of-plane and therefore cross-sectional view of the vein. (*B*) In-plane and therefore longitudinal view of the vein.

visualization, and was found to have a higher success rate for internal jugular vein cannulations compared with short-axis or long-axis approaches.[32]

With any of these approaches, the skin puncture point of the needle should be close to the probe, and at an angle of 30° to 45°. Once the needle is in the vein, the probe can be released to facilitate threading of the guidewire. The position of the guidewire can be confirmed by scanning the course of the vein and identifying a hyperechoic artifact within the lumen of the vein, which adds the benefit of confirming the vein and guidewire position before dilatation of the vessel.

In a similar method, arterial cannulation can be facilitated under ultrasonographic guidance. Sites that can typically be used with ultrasonography include the radial, brachial, and femoral arteries. Once again, in-plane or out-of-plane techniques can be used, as long as the clinician becomes familiar with the ultrasonographic appearances of arteries and the nearby anatomy.

Difficult peripheral venous cannulation can also be guided under real-time ultrasonography, and the deep veins of the forearm are particularly amenable to this procedure.

Cricothyroid Membrane Identification

Nature of the problem
Identification of the cricothyroid membrane is a critical skill for all anesthesiologists. It allows emergency cricothyrotomy to be performed, which may be lifesaving in the context of a cannot-intubate, cannot-oxygenate crisis. However, this skill is infrequently practiced and thus the identification of the cricothyroid membrane among anesthesiologists may be poor. A major airway study from the United Kingdom has shown an alarmingly high rate of failure of cricothyrotomy by anesthesiologists.[33]

A recent investigation comparing the success rate of cricothyrotomy in cadavers with difficult anatomic landmarks has shown an almost 6-fold increase in success rate and a lower rate of injuries with ultrasonography facilitation versus palpation identification.[34] In another study, in women of childbearing age, palpation of the cricothyroid membrane proved to be poor, and increasingly difficult in obese women.[35] When laboring women were studied, identification of the cricothyroid membrane by palpation was correct in only 71% and 39% of nonobese and obese parturients respectively. Although it is clear that obesity makes palpation of anatomic landmarks difficult, the investigators concluded that ultrasonography visualization of the cricothyroid membrane in the setting of increased adipose tissue is not difficult.[36]

Indications for cricothyroid membrane ultrasonography
Performing ultrasonography to delineate the cricothyroid membrane is a fairly new concept. The investigators of the 4th National Audit Project (NAP4) study stressed the need to plan for airway failure by developing a strategy involving a logical sequence of steps from the onset, if a potential difficult airway is suspected.[33] Given the higher risk of airway complexities in the obstetric population, and the increasing incidence of obesity compromising rescue efforts, obstetric anesthesiologists should be adequately prepared to address a cannot-intubate, cannot-oxygenate emergent scenario.

Preemptive marking of the cricothyroid membrane in the suspected troublesome airway, caused by either abnormal anatomy or obesity, can be helpful. This marking could be done before operative delivery either with planned regional or general anesthesia. In addition, if there is a laboring parturient with a concerning airway, the clinician could proactively use ultrasonography to mark the airway in case of prospective emergencies, which are common in the delivery suite.

Technique

Identification of the cricothyroid membrane is undertaken with the patient supine. The neck should be extended and this positioning duly noted. If cricothyrotomy is subsequently required, it should be performed in exactly the same position as the ultrasonography.

With palpation, locate the sternal notch, and place a linear probe in a transverse position directly superior to the sternal notch. The trachea, a large hypoechoic structure with a surrounding hyperechoic rim, is visualized in the center. Proceed to move the probe laterally to the patient's right side, until the trachea is seen only at the left side of the screen. The probe should be swiveled 90° anticlockwise and held in a longitudinal plane (**Fig. 15**A). A hyperechoic bright line is seen, which represents the tissue-air border of the anterior surface of the airway. Superficial to this line, a series of small circular hypoechoic structures are seen, analogous to a string of pearls. These structures represent the individual tracheal rings.

As the probe is moved more cephalad, the string of pearls terminates with a larger ovoid hypoechoic structure, the cricoid cartilage (**Fig. 15**B, C). The area directly cephalad to this structure is the cricothyroid membrane, which can then be marked.

CURRENT CONTROVERSIES/FUTURE CONSIDERATIONS

The use of ultrasonography for central vascular access is well established, with a steep learning curve for novices. However, performing proficient ultrasonography of

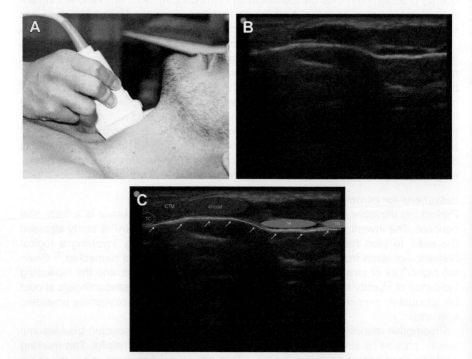

Fig. 15. Cricothyroid membrane ultrasonography. (*A*) Longitudinal placement of the probe. (*B, C*) Corresponding sonoanatomy, showing cricothyroid membrane, cricoid, tracheal rings, and anterior tracheal wall. Arrows indicate the tissue-air border of the anterior tracheal wall. CTM, cricothyroid membrane; TC, thyroid cartilage; TR, tracheal ring.

the spine, lung, or stomach requires a level of training for which the learning curve is yet to be identified. For spinal ultrasonography, after teaching with reading material, a video presentation, a 45-minute didactic lecture, and a 30-minute hands-on workshop, novices were unable to show full transfer of knowledge and competence.[37] With regard to learning gastric ultrasonography, a group of novice anesthesiologists receiving formal teaching as well as an interactive 3-hour hands-on workshop were found to require approximately 33 gastric examinations to achieve a 95% qualitative assessment success rate, as determined by a predictive model.[38] The nature of the effective methods and volume of cases required for full transfer of knowledge for novices to achieve competence and proficiency in ultrasonography for various applications remains to be determined. Furthermore, expertise in ultrasonography is gained by repetitive scanning in routine cases, rather than by using it reservedly for difficult cases.

Although real-time ultrasonography for central vascular access and peripheral nerve blockade is recommended and feasible in maintaining direct vision of the needle, using a similar technique for neuraxial block remains a challenge. Spinal ultrasonography is performed preprocedure to locate the desired interspace and optimal puncture point, facilitate the angle of insertion, and estimate the depth to the epidural space. Performing neuraxial anesthesia under real-time ultrasonography has proved to be technically challenging for several reasons, including the need for an assistant to perform the ultrasonography or the loss of resistance technique, and the maintenance of meticulous sterility. Epidural insertion under real-time ultrasonography has been described,[39] but this is still a novel practice.

Although the use of ultrasonography in anesthesia is well established, it still remains a fairly new tool in the armamentarium. Despite the development of protocols for gastric and lung ultrasonography, its direct role in clinical care in the labor and delivery suite remains to be established. Gastric and lung ultrasonography in the obstetric cohort is in its infancy, and further research for inter-rater reliability, feasibility, and implications for clinical care need to be addressed. Furthermore, the exact role of ultrasonography-facilitated preemptive marking of the cricothyroid membrane in an unanticipated cannot-intubate, cannot-oxygenate crisis has yet to be defined. Spinal ultrasonography is more recognized in its use, and the benefits are clear. More convincing are the benefits of ultrasonography facilitation for central vascular access and peripheral nerve blocks; few anesthesiologists perform these procedures without ultrasonography guidance if possible.

The future scope of ultrasonography in obstetric anesthesia includes the use of echocardiography and, possibly, optic nerve sheath scanning. Echocardiography no longer remains a specific skill of cardiologists. Intensive care physicians and anesthesiologists have embraced this highly desirable artistry and it could be easily transferable to the labor and delivery suite. In addition, serial scanning of the optic nerve sheath diameter may be a desirable tool to estimate the degree of cerebral edema and guide clinical management in preeclamptic patients. The optic nerve sheath diameter has been shown to be a reliable surrogate detector of intracranial hypertension.[40] The triennial maternal mortality report from the United Kingdom has repeatedly shown neurologic disease as a significant contributor to peripartum mortality, and has mandated full neurologic assessment in all women with new headaches or atypical symptoms.[41] Investigators have shown that 20% of preeclamptic patients examined with optic nerve sheath ultrasonography have findings that correlate with intracranial pressures greater than 20 mm Hg.[42]

SUMMARY

The applications of ultrasonography in obstetric anesthesia are growing and the potential use of this tool to facilitate the clinical management of pregnant patients is increasing. The learning curves for full transfer of knowledge of ultrasonography competencies is uncertain, and some applications for routine practice are yet to be determined. However, the increased safety, enhanced accuracy in diagnosis, and improved efficacy for interventions with ultrasonography in obstetric anesthesia cannot be ignored.

REFERENCES

1. National Institute for Clinical Excellence. Guidance on the use of ultrasound locating devices for placing central venous catheters. National Institute for Clinical Excellence; 2002. Available at: http://www.nice.org.uk. Accessed October 31, 2016.
2. Rupp SM, Apfelbaum JL, Blitt C, et al. Practice guidelines for central venous access: a report by the American Society of Anesthesiologists Task Force on Central Venous Access. Anesthesiology 2012;116:539–73.
3. National Institute for Clinical Excellence. Ultrasound-guided regional nerve block. National Institute for Clinical Excellence; 2009. Available at: http://www.nice.org.uk. Accessed October 31, 2016.
4. Kurinczuk J, Churchill D, Cox P, et al. Messages for the care of women who died between six weeks and a year after pregnancy. In: Knight M, Tuffnell D, Kenyon S, on behalf of MBBRACE-UK, et al, editors. Saving lives, improving mothers' care - surveillance of maternal deaths in the UK 2011-13 and lessons learned to inform maternity care from the UK and Ireland confidential enquiries into maternal deaths and morbidity 2009-13. Oxford (United Kingdom): National Perinatal Epidemiology Unit; University of Oxford; 2015. p. 71–81.
5. Broadbent CR, Maxwell WB, Ferrie R, et al. Ability of anaesthetists to identify a marked lumbar interspace. Anaesthesia 2000;55:1122–6.
6. Grau T, Bartusseck E, Conradi R, et al. Ultrasound imaging improves learning curves in obstetric epidural anesthesia: a preliminary study. Can J Anesth 2003;50:1047–50.
7. Shaikh F, Brzezinski J, Alexander S, et al. Ultrasound imaging for lumbar punctures and epidural catheterisations: systematic review and meta-analysis. BMJ 2013;346:f1720.
8. National Institute for Clinical Excellence. Ultrasound-guided catheterization of the epidural space. National Institute for Clinical Excellence; 2009. Available at: http://www.nice.org.uk. Accessed October 31, 2016.
9. Chin KJ, Perlas A, Chan V, et al. Ultrasound imaging facilitates spinal anesthesia in adults with difficult surface anatomic landmarks. Anesthesiology 2011;115:94–101.
10. Carvalho JC. Ultrasound-facilitated epidurals and spinals in obstetrics. Anesthesiol Clin 2008;26:145–58.
11. Mendelson CL. The aspiration of stomach contents into the lungs during obstetric anesthesia. Am J Obstet Gynecol 1946;52:191–205.
12. Cubillos J, Tse C, Chan VW, et al. Bedside ultrasound assessment of gastric content: an observational study. Can J Anesth 2012;59(4):416–23.
13. Levy DM. Pre-operative fasting—60 years on from Mendelson. Contin Educ Anaesth Crit Care Pain 2006;6:215–8.
14. Chiloiro M, Darconza G, Piccioli E, et al. Gastric emptying and orocecal transit time in pregnancy. J Gastroenterol 2001;36:538–43.

15. Wong CA, Loffredi M, Ganchiff JN, et al. Gastric emptying of water in term pregnancy. Anesthesiology 2002;96:1395–400.
16. Wong CA, McCarthy RJ, Fitzgerald PC, et al. Gastric emptying of water in obese pregnant women at term. Anesth Analg 2007;105:751–5.
17. Carp H, Jayaram A, Stoll M. Ultrasound examination of the stomach contents of parturients. Anesth Analg 1992;74:683–7.
18. Bataille A, Rousset J, Marret E, et al. Ultrasonographic evaluation of gastric content during labour under epidural analgesia: a prospective cohort study. Br J Anaesth 2014;112:703–7.
19. Kubli M, Scrutton MJ, Seed PT, et al. An evaluation of isotonic "sport drinks" during labor. Anesth Analg 2002;94:404–8.
20. Van de Putte P, Perlas A. Ultrasound assessment of gastric content and volume. Br J Anaesth 2014;113:12–22.
21. Dennis AT, Solnordal CB. Acute pulmonary oedema in pregnant women. Anaesthesia 2012;67:646–59.
22. Volpicelli G, Elbarbary M, Blaivas M, et al. International evidence-based recommendations for point-of-care lung ultrasound. Intensive Care Med 2012;38:577–91.
23. Noble VE, Lamhaut L, Capp R, et al. Evaluation of a thoracic ultrasound training module for the detection of pneumothorax and pulmonary edema by prehospital physician care providers. BMC Med Educ 2009;9:1.
24. Zieleskiewicz L, Lagier D, Contargyris C, et al. Lung ultrasound-guided management of acute breathlessness during pregnancy. Anaesthesia 2013;68:97–101.
25. McDonnell JG, Curley G, Carney J, et al. The analgesic efficacy of transversus abdominis plane block after cesarean delivery: a randomized controlled trial. Anesth Analg 2008;106:186–91.
26. McDermott G, Korba E, Mata U, et al. Should we stop doing blind transversus abdominis plane blocks? Br J Anaesth 2012;108:499–502.
27. Farooq M, Carey M. A case of liver trauma with a blunt regional anesthesia needle while performing transversus abdominis plane block. Reg Anesth Pain Med 2008;33:274–5.
28. Baeriswyl M, Kirkham KR, Kern C, et al. The analgesic efficacy of ultrasound-guided transversus abdominis plane block in adult patients: a meta-analysis. Anesth Analg 2015;121:1640–54.
29. Belavy D, Cowlishaw PJ, Howes M, et al. Ultrasound-guided transversus abdominis plane block for analgesia after Caesarean delivery. Br J Anaesth 2009;103:726–30.
30. Abdallah FW, Halpern SH, Margarido CB. Transversus abdominis plane block for postoperative analgesia after Caesarean delivery performed under spinal anesthesia? A systematic review and meta-analysis. Br J Anaesth 2012;109:679–87.
31. Brass P, Hellmich M, Kolodziej L, et al. Ultrasound guidance versus anatomical landmarks for internal jugular vein catheterization. Cochrane Database Syst Rev 2015;(1):CD006962.
32. Batllori M, Urra M, Uriarte E, et al. Randomized comparison of three transducer orientation approaches for ultrasound guided internal jugular venous cannulation. Br J Anaesth 2016;116:370–6.
33. Cook TM, Woodall N, Frerk CO. Major complications of airway management in the UK: results of the Fourth National Audit Project of the Royal College of Anaesthetists and the Difficult Airway Society. Part 1: anaesthesia. Br J Anaesth 2011;106:617–31.

34. Siddiqui N, Arzola C, Friedman Z, et al. Ultrasound improves cricothyrotomy success in cadavers with poorly defined neck anatomy. A Randomized Control Trial. Anesthesiology 2015;123:1033–41.

35. Aslani A, Ng SC, Hurley M, et al. Accuracy of identification of the cricothyroid membrane in female subjects using palpation: an observational study. Anesth Analg 2012;114:987–92.

36. You-Ten KE, Desai D, Postonogova T, et al. Accuracy of conventional digital palpation and ultrasound of the cricothyroid membrane in obese women in labour. Anaesthesia 2015;70:1230–4.

37. Margarido CB, Arzola C, Balki M, et al. Anesthesiologists' learning curves for ultrasound assessment of the lumbar spine. Can J Anesth 2010;57:120–6.

38. Arzola C, Carvalho JC, Cubillos J, et al. Anesthesiologists' learning curves for bedside qualitative ultrasound assessment of gastric content: a cohort study. Can J Anesth 2013;60:771–9.

39. Karmakar MK, Li X, Ho AM, et al. Real-time ultrasound guided paramedian epidural access: evaluation of a novel in-plane technique. Br J Anaesth 2009; 102:845–54.

40. Dubourg J, Javouhey E, Geeraerts T, et al. Ultrasonography of optic nerve sheath diameter for detection of raised intracranial pressure: a systematic review and meta-analysis. Intensive Care Med 2011;37:1059–68.

41. Kemp B, MacKillop L, Yoong A, et al. Caring for women with cancer in pregnancy or postpartum. In: Knight M, Tuffnell D, Kenyon S, on behalf of MBBRACE-UK, et al, editors. Saving lives, improving mothers' care - surveillance of maternal deaths in the UK 2011-13 and lessons learned to inform maternity care from the UK and Ireland confidential enquiries into maternal deaths and morbidity 2009-13. Oxford (United Kingdom): National Perinatal Epidemiology Unit; University of Oxford; 2015. p. 53–61.

42. Dubost C, Le Gouez A, Jouffroy V, et al. Optic nerve sheath diameter used as ultrasonographic assessment of the incidence of raised intracranial pressure in preeclampsia: a pilot study. Anesthesiology 2012;116:1066–71.

Huddles and Debriefings

Improving Communication on Labor and Delivery

Emily McQuaid-Hanson, MD*, May C.M. Pian-Smith, MD

KEYWORDS

- Preoperative huddle • Postoperative debriefing • Adverse event debriefing
- Patient safety • Obstetric anesthesia

KEY POINTS

- Benefits of preoperative huddles include improvements in patient safety, efficiency, communication, and teamwork.
- Preoperative huddles are effective and important in a wide variety of clinical settings, but are particularly well suited to labor and delivery.
- Postoperative debriefing after routine cases allows for ongoing learning, process improvement, and improvements in teamwork.
- Postoperative debriefing after an adverse event benefits both patients and providers and helps prevent the "second victim" phenomenon.

INTRODUCTION

The labor and delivery unit is a unique and dynamic environment. Add-on cases, schedule changes, emergency surgeries—features that are relatively rare and contained in a hospital's main operating suite—are routine on labor and delivery. Patients' conditions evolve constantly and change unexpectedly. Such an environment poses unique challenges and rewards for the anesthesiologist and all members of the care team. Communication between and among team members is essential to maintain patient safety as well as to prevent provider frustration and burnout.

Preoperative huddles and postoperative debriefings have been shown to be valuable across a wide variety of medical and surgical environments.[1–6] Benefits of huddles include improved patient safety, decreased incidence of preventable errors, increased efficiency, and promotion and continued development of a multidisciplinary

Departments of Anesthesia, Critical Care, and Pain Medicine, Harvard Medical School, Massachusetts General Hospital, 55 Fruit Street, Jackson 440, Boston, MA 02114, USA
* Corresponding author.
E-mail address: emcquaid-hanson@mgh.harvard.edu

Anesthesiology Clin 35 (2017) 59–67
http://dx.doi.org/10.1016/j.anclin.2016.09.006
1932-2275/17/© 2016 Elsevier Inc. All rights reserved.

care team model of patient care. Postoperative debriefings may occur either on a routine basis or in the setting of an adverse event. Benefits of routine postoperative debriefings are similar to those of the huddle, but also extend to process and quality improvement through retrospective knowledge of clinical issues and prompt identification of issues with systems or equipment. Debriefings that occur after an adverse event take a somewhat different form, and confer some overlapping, but also some unique benefits. Costs associated with implementing and adhering to huddle and debriefing systems are minimal, especially when weighed against the potential for patient harm when they are not used. In this article, the authors explore the history of preoperative huddles and related procedures, define huddles and debriefings and their potential components and participants, and discuss the benefits and drawbacks associated with their use. They also discuss some of the benefits of huddles and debriefings that make them uniquely well suited to the labor and delivery unit.

HISTORICAL PERSPECTIVE

The concept of a huddle was initially borrowed from the world of football. In 1894, Paul D. Hubbard was the quarterback at Gallaudet University, an institution for the deaf and hard of hearing in Washington, DC. Hubbard is credited with inventing the huddle. By bringing his teammates together in a tightly formed circle, he was able to communicate key information about the upcoming play using sign language, without revealing his strategy to the opposing team.[7,8] The circular formation allowed for eye contact between team members, clear communication, privacy, and minimized distractions. The huddle has since been widely adopted in professional football and other sports. The exact point at which the technique was adopted into medicine is unclear; however, references start to appear in the literature as early as 1993.[9] By the mid-2000s, the use of huddles in medical practice was being widely studied and described in multiple fields, most notably in the operating room and surgical subspecialties.[1,10,11] The publication of Atul Gawande's New Yorker article, "The Checklist" in 2007, and his subsequent nonfiction bestseller The Checklist Manifesto,[12,13] further heightened public awareness of the importance of process improvement to prevent medical errors and inspired additional research studies.

Interest in debriefings followed a similar trajectory throughout the first decade of this century, as the medical community focused on the importance of communication among medical professionals in improving patient safety and reducing provider stress and burnout. At the national level, organizations such as the Joint Commission implicated communication breakdown as a root cause in 50% to 70% of sentinel events,[14,15] resulting in serious patient morbidity and mortality. At the global level, the World Health Organization introduced a suite of interventions in 2009, aimed at making surgery safer. This suite of interventions included the Surgical Safety Checklist, preoperative briefings, and postoperative debriefings.[16] Altogether, there has been increasing emphasis placed on the role of high-level teamwork, communication, and situational awareness in protecting the safety of patients and improving the happiness and productivity of providers. Further research and developments in this area can be anticipated in the coming years.

THE PREOPERATIVE HUDDLE ON LABOR AND DELIVERY: WHO, WHAT, WHEN, AND WHERE?

The huddle is a briefing that takes place among providers shortly before the start of a procedure, with the purpose of sharing information, coordinating care, and providing an opportunity for members of the care team to raise safety concerns. There are no set rules about who is involved, what information is included, or where the huddle occurs: the information presented herein represents some of a wide variety of possibilities.

Who: Commonly described participants in the preoperative huddle include the following:

- Surgeons/obstetricians
- Anesthesia providers
- Bedside nursing staff
- Operating room nursing staff/scrub technician
- The patient

Additional participants on labor and delivery may include midwives, labor doulas, and neonatal intensive care unit staff.[17,18]

What: Components of the huddle are highly variable, but commonly incorporated information includes the following:

- Team introductions and statement of roles
- Confirmation of patient identity, signed consent forms, and allergies
- Surgery or procedure to be performed, site marking if applicable
- Urgency of surgery or procedure
- Critical and nonroutine steps of the surgery or procedure
- Availability and readiness of implants/special equipment
- Review of pertinent laboratory values
- Anticipated blood loss and availability/need for uterotonics or blood products
- Planned anesthetic and monitoring, and airway and other anesthetic concerns
- Neonatal concerns
- Antibiotic administration/dosing
- Deep venous thrombosis prophylaxis
- Postoperative disposition
- Additional concerns

Some institutions make use of a checklist or other cognitive aid in their preoperative huddles. Potential advantages of a checklist are decreased risk of forgetting a component, and that the presence of the list itself may serve as a reminder to perform the huddle. These advantages are not insignificant, given that studies of huddle implementation show that compliance can be poor, especially when the practice is first introduced.[19] There is also evidence that routine use of a checklist improves communication and recall of critical steps in situations in which performing a huddle is not possible, such as a STAT cesarean delivery.[17] Potential disadvantages are decreased flexibility in the type and order of information covered, impaired ability to think "outside the box" when dictated by an evolving clinical situation, as well as the risk that team members may perceive the checklist as overly rigid or rote,[18] and therefore, be less engaged in the process.

Where: The exact location of the huddle is less important than the qualities of the environment. The huddle may take place in or outside of the patient's room, in the operating room, or in another convenient location. Choosing a location that minimizes noise pollution and other distractions is important to facilitate clear communication and improve focus.[20]

THE WHY: BENEFITS OF PREOPERATIVE HUDDLES

The benefits of huddles have been demonstrated in obstetrics and across a wide range of surgical specialties.

Patient Safety

Studies have shown that huddles result in a higher percentage of on-time administration of perioperative antibiotics and deep vein thrombosis prophylaxis[2,21] as well as reducing the number of unanticipated events or "near misses" in the operating room.[20]

Efficiency

Huddles do not delay operating room start times,[22] and in some situations they have been shown to increase the percentage of on-time or early starts.[11,23,24] Huddles have also been shown to decrease unanticipated events related to equipment[20,25] and improve surgeons' perceptions of work flow.[6]

Communication and Teamwork

Huddles have been shown to improve communication between team members[10,22,26] and internal perceptions of teamwork.[1,20,24] Improved communication is achieved through several mechanisms, including by providing a framework that circumvents the traditional hierarchical structure of the operating room,[22] creating a designated, protected time in which to share information and ask questions, and through standardizing and ensuring uniformity of language.[26] Huddles can improve communication between nursing staff and surgeons as well as interdisciplinary communication between specialties, for example, between surgeons and anesthesiologists,[1,10] or between obstetricians and neonatologists.[17] Interestingly, implementation of a preoperative huddle has also been shown to improve the accuracy of team members' self-assessment of teamwork behavior. Their self-assessments more closely match peer assessments, as opposed to being more favorable than those from their peers.[27]

Accountability and Speaking Up

Huddles enhance team members' sense of accountability and empowerment[26] and make it easier to speak up.[19,22] This effect is most pronounced for nurses and other team members who are traditionally perceived as occupying a lower status in the operating room hierarchy. Empowering team members and patients to speak up has been identified by organizations such as the Joint Commission and the Institute of Medicine as a critical step in improving patient safety and avoiding adverse outcomes.[28,29] The preoperative huddle promotes and facilitates this process by providing a place and a time in which all team members are not only allowed, but encouraged to raise concerns.

THE WHY NOT: DRAWBACKS OF PREOPERATIVE HUDDLES

Most of the barriers to implementing a preoperative briefing can broadly be categorized in 1 of 2 ways: logistical and cultural. The logistical barriers primarily relate to time, most notably persistent fears that huddles will contribute to surgical delays. Evidence suggests that huddles either have no impact on surgical start times or increase the percentage of on-time starts,[11,22,24] and that an effective huddle can be accomplished in as little as 1 minute.[6] However, there is certainly overhead cost involved in the form of planning, materials, and staff training. No direct financial analyses exist regarding the costs of implementing a preoperative huddle. Given the high cost of operating room time and adverse patient outcomes such as wound infections and deep vein thromboses, the potential financial benefits most likely outweigh the costs of implementation.

As compared with logistic obstacles, cultural barriers are likely more tenacious and difficult to either disprove or circumnavigate. The collaborative and antihierarchical nature of the huddle may challenge physician team members' sense of autonomy and authority,[19] and other team members can become frustrated by lack of buy-in from their surgical colleagues. In certain situations, huddles have been shown to reinforce, rather than transcend, existing interprofessional hierarchies.[30] These and other studies highlight the importance of strong leadership[31] and up-front multidisciplinary collaboration when implementing these changes.

LEARNING AND PROCESSING: POSTOPERATIVE DEBRIEFINGS

The routine postoperative debriefing is a brief review that occurs at the conclusion of an operation. The goal of debriefing is to reflect on both negative and positive events that occurred during the case while it is still vivid in the minds of the team members as well as to identify and promptly address issues regarding equipment or processes. It may also serve as a time to coordinate care and plan for the ongoing needs of the current patient in the operating room.[25]

Many of the benefits of postoperative debriefings mimic those of the preoperative huddle, such as enhancing communication and teamwork,[32,33] and indeed the 2 interventions are often implemented and studied simultaneously. The postoperative debriefing typically involves the same complement of team members as the preoperative huddle. It typically takes place in the operating room immediately after the surgery ends, or even while it is still ongoing, for example, during skin closure. Like the preoperative huddle, the postoperative debriefing may make use of a checklist or cognitive aid. Items included in the postoperative debriefing include the following:

- Summary of procedure, including totals for blood loss, urine output, intravenous fluids, blood products, and medications administered
- Labeling of pathologic specimens with correct patient information
- "What went well/what could have gone better?"
- Communication/safety concerns
- Equipment issues
- Efficiency issues
- Transition of care/postoperative planning

One benefit that is unique to postoperative briefing is the ability for the operating room team to engage in active, ongoing process improvement. Problems, such as those with surgical equipment, are immediately identified and potentially addressed in real time. These actions may not only improve patient safety and outcomes[2,34,35] but also have the potential to contribute significantly to operating room efficiency.[33,34,36] The act of reflection has been shown to be a key component of adult learning,[37,38] suggesting that implementing a postoperative debriefing is likely to elevate the performance and effectiveness of operating room staff. The ability to highlight accomplishments and commend team members for a job well done is also unique to the debriefing process[38,39] and has the potential to have a profound effect on morale, reinforce a sense of teamwork, and improve job satisfaction.[5]

PREVENTING THE SECOND VICTIM: DEBRIEFING AFTER ADVERSE EVENTS

Adverse medical events not only affect patients but also have been shown to have serious psychological impact on health care providers.[40] The term "second victim" has been used to recognize the traumatic effects that can be experienced by the practitioners who are involved in such adverse events.[41] Another layer of the second victim concept relates to the patients who are cared for *after* the event, whose care may be impacted or influenced by the distress, distraction, and loss of confidence of their providers.[40,42] Debriefing after an adverse event has been shown to make participants feel more supported by their colleagues,[43] facilitate adult learning and processing of information,[37] and improve subsequent performance on both an individual and a team level.[44–46] Debriefing may also facilitate providers' consistency and cohesiveness when interacting with patients after an adverse event, which is important because the quality and effectiveness of communication impact patients' perceptions of the event as well as their satisfaction with their care.[47]

Debriefings that occur following an adverse event share many features with the routine postoperative debriefings, but they also have some unique features. Adverse event debriefings occur hours to weeks after an event. The key participants in these debriefings are the team members who were involved in the case either directly (nurses, obstetricians, anesthesiologists, neonatologists) or indirectly (eg, pathologists, radiologists, resource managers). However, involvement of a variety of additional personnel may also be appropriate, including unit or departmental leaders, risk management or patient advocacy representatives, and psychological services. The format of the adverse event debriefing is typically fluid and conversational as opposed to rigidly scripted; however, strong leadership is important not only to guide the discussion but also to set a tone that will minimize blame, facilitate communication, encourage participation, and enhance learning.[44,48,49]

TWO PATIENTS AND CONSTANT CHANGES: HUDDLES AND DEBRIEFINGS ON LABOR AND DELIVERY

The labor and delivery unit is a uniquely challenging and rewarding medical environment. A patient's status is inherently dynamic and constantly evolving, and every parturient represents 2 patients. A truly multidisciplinary, multispecialty team of providers is involved in the care of each patient, with the potential for conflicting goals. Most of the patients on labor and delivery are fully awake and aware throughout all procedures; family members are frequently present, and the nature of the situation lends itself to heightened emotions and anxiety for everyone involved.

For these and other reasons, establishing the culture and tradition of preoperative huddles and postoperative debriefings is important on the labor and delivery unit. The Joint Commission performed a root cause analysis of sentinel perinatal events leading to mortality or permanent disability, which included 47 cases between 1996 and 2004.[14] The leading identified root cause was communication breakdown (72%), with more than half of the involved parties citing cultural barriers such as hierarchy, intimidation, and failure to function as a team as specific contributing factors. Such data highlight the critical importance of huddles and debriefings, because these interventions have been shown not only to improve communication but also to address the cultural issues that have been identified as contributing to these events.[50] Although implementation of huddles and debriefings appears to be a relatively simple step, the scope of their impact should not be ignored: the potential for happier, healthier, and safer deliveries for our patients and their infants.

REFERENCES

1. Makary MA, Mukherjee A, Sexton JB, et al. Operating room briefings and wrong-site surgery. J Am Coll Surg 2007;204(2):236–43.

2. Paull DE, Mazzia LM, Wood SD, et al. Briefing guide study: preoperative briefing and postoperative debriefing checklists in the Veterans Health Administration medical team training program. Am J Surg 2010;200(5):620–3.

3. Muething SE, Goudie A, Schoettker PJ, et al. Quality improvement initiative to reduce serious safety events and improve patient safety culture. Pediatrics 2012;130(2):e423–31.
4. Brady PW, Muething S, Kotagal U, et al. Improving situation awareness to reduce unrecognized clinical deterioration and serious safety events. Pediatrics 2013; 131(1):e298–308.
5. Hill MR, Roberts MJ, Alderson ML, et al. Safety culture and the 5 steps to safer surgery: an intervention study. Br J Anaesth 2015;114(6):958–62.
6. Jain AL, Jones KC, Simon J, et al. The impact of a daily pre-operative surgical huddle on interruptions, delays, and surgeon satisfaction in an orthopedic operating room: a prospective study. Patient Saf Surg 2015;9:8.
7. Gannon J. Deaf heritage: a narrative of deaf America. Silver Spring (MD): National Association of the Deaf; 1981.
8. Glymph DC, Olenick M, Barbera S, et al. Healthcare utilizing deliberate discussion linking events (HUDDLE): a systematic review. AANA J 2015;83(3):183–8.
9. Nacht ES. 14 Ingredients of "the huddle" in the practice of pediatric dentistry. J Clin Pediatr Dent 1993;17(4):211–2.
10. Awad SS, Fagan SP, Bellows C, et al. Bridging the communication gap in the operating room with medical team training. Am J Surg 2005;190(5):770–4.
11. Nundy S, Mukherjee A, Sexton JB, et al. Impact of preoperative briefings on operating room delays: a preliminary report. Arch Surg 2008;143(11):1068–72.
12. Gawande A. The Checklist. The New Yorker 2007.
13. Gawande A. The checklist manifesto: how to get things right. New York: Metropolitan Books; 2009.
14. Preventing infant death and injury during delivery. Jt Comm Perspect 2004;24(9): 14–5.
15. Sentinel Event Data: Root Causes by Event Type 2004-2013. Joint Commission on Accreditation of Healthcare Organizations. Available at: https://www.jointcommission.org/sentinel_event.aspx. Accessed November 22, 2016.
16. World Health Organization. Guidelines for Safer Surgery. Geneva (Switzerland): World Health Organization; 2009. Available at: http://www.who.int/patientsafety/safesurgery/tools_resources/9789241598552/en/. Accessed November 22, 2016.
17. Dadiz R, Weinschreider J, Schriefer J, et al. Interdisciplinary simulation-based training to improve delivery room communication. Simul Healthc 2013;8(5): 279–91.
18. Kacmar R, editor. Every woman who delivers by cesarean deserves a pre-operative huddle, in SOAP Patient Safety Committee "How We Do It" Expert Opinion. Society for Obstetric Anesthesia and Perinatology. Available at: https://soap.org/expert-opinions-every-woman.php. Accessed November 22, 2016.
19. Khoshbin A, Lingard L, Wright JG. Evaluation of preoperative and perioperative operating room briefings at the Hospital for Sick Children. Can J Surg 2009; 52(4):309–15.
20. Einav Y, Gopher D, Kara I, et al. Preoperative briefing in the operating room: shared cognition, teamwork, and patient safety. Chest 2010;137(2):443–9.
21. Lingard L, Regehr G, Cartmill C, et al. Evaluation of a preoperative team briefing: a new communication routine results in improved clinical practice. BMJ Qual Saf 2011;20(6):475–82.
22. Ali M, Osborne A, Bethune R, et al. Preoperative surgical briefings do not delay operating room start times and are popular with surgical team members. J Patient Saf 2011;7(3):139–43.

23. Wright JG, Roche A, Khoury AE. Improving on-time surgical starts in an operating room. Can J Surg 2010;53(3):167–70.

24. Bethune R, Sasirekha G, Sahu A, et al. Use of briefings and debriefings as a tool in improving team work, efficiency, and communication in the operating theatre. Postgrad Med J 2011;87(1027):331–4.

25. Papaspyros SC, Javangula KC, Adluri RK, et al. Briefing and debriefing in the cardiac operating room. Analysis of impact on theatre team attitude and patient safety. Interact Cardiovasc Thorac Surg 2010;10(1):43–7.

26. Goldenhar LM, Brady PW, Sutcliffe KM, et al. Huddling for high reliability and situation awareness. BMJ Qual Saf 2013;22(11):899–906.

27. Paige JT, Aaron DL, Yang T, et al. Implementation of a preoperative briefing protocol improves accuracy of teamwork assessment in the operating room. Am Surg 2008;74(9):817–23.

28. Sentinel events: evaluating cause and planning improvement. 2nd edition. Oakbrook Terrace (IL): Joint Commission on Accreditation of Healthcare Organizations; 1998.

29. Committee on Quality of Health Care in America. To err is human: building a safer health system. In: Kohn LT, Corrigan JM, Donaldson MS, editors. Creating safety systems in health care organizations. Washington, DC: Institute of Medicine; 1999. p. 102–55.

30. Whyte S, Cartmill C, Gardezi F, et al. Uptake of a team briefing in the operating theatre: a Burkean dramatistic analysis. Soc Sci Med 2009;69(12):1757–66.

31. Paull DE, Mazzia LM, Izu BS, et al. Predictors of successful implementation of preoperative briefings and postoperative debriefings after medical team training. Am J Surg 2009;198(5):675–8.

32. Berenholtz SM, Schumacher K, Hayanga AJ, et al. Implementing standardized operating room briefings and debriefings at a large regional medical center. Jt Comm J Qual Patient Saf 2009;35(8):391–7.

33. Wolf FA, Way LW, Stewart L. The efficacy of medical team training: improved team performance and decreased operating room delays: a detailed analysis of 4863 cases. Ann Surg 2010;252(3):477–83 [discussion: 483–5].

34. Weiner E, Bar J, Fainstein N, et al. The effect of a program to shorten the decision-to-delivery interval for emergent cesarean section on maternal and neonatal outcome. Am J Obstet Gynecol 2014;210(3):224.e1-6.

35. Zuckerman SL, France DJ, Green C, et al. Surgical debriefing: a reliable roadmap to completing the patient safety cycle. Neurosurg Focus 2012;33(5):E4.

36. Porta CR, Foster A, Causey MW, et al. Operating room efficiency improvement after implementation of a postoperative team assessment. J Surg Res 2013; 180(1):15–20.

37. McGreevy JM, Otten TD. Briefing and debriefing in the operating room using fighter pilot crew resource management. J Am Coll Surg 2007;205(1):169–76.

38. Ahmed M, Sevdalis N, Paige J, et al. Identifying best practice guidelines for debriefing in surgery: a tri-continental study. Am J Surg 2012;203(4):523–9.

39. Miller KK, Riley W, Davis S, et al. In situ simulation: a method of experiential learning to promote safety and team behavior. J Perinat Neonatal Nurs 2008; 22(2):105–13.

40. Waterman AD, Garbutt J, Hazel E, et al. The emotional impact of medical errors on practicing physicians in the United States and Canada. Jt Comm J Qual Patient Saf 2007;33(8):467–76.

41. Scott SD, Hirschinger LE, Cox KR, et al. The natural history of recovery for the healthcare provider "second victim" after adverse patient events. Qual Saf Health Care 2009;18(5):325–30.

42. Bognar A, Barach P, Johnson JK, et al. Errors and the burden of errors: attitudes, perceptions, and the culture of safety in pediatric cardiac surgical teams. Ann Thorac Surg 2008;85(4):1374–81.

43. Tan H. Debriefing after critical incidents for anaesthetic trainees. Anaesth Intensive Care 2005;33(6):768–72.

44. McDonnell LK, JK, Dismukes RK. Facilitation LOS debriefings: a training manual, in NASA Technical memorandum. 1997.Available at: https://www.faa.gov/training_testing/training/aqp/library/media/Final_Training_TM.pdf. Accessed November 22, 2016.

45. Mathieu JE, Heffner TS, Goodwin GF, et al. The influence of shared mental models on team process and performance. J Appl Psychol 2000;85(2):273–83.

46. Darling M, Parry C, Moore J. Learning in the thick of it. Harv Bus Rev 2005;83(7): 84–92, 192.

47. Duclos CW, Eichler M, Taylor L, et al. Patient perspectives of patient-provider communication after adverse events. Int J Qual Health Care 2005;17(6):479–86.

48. Rudolph JW, Simon R, Rivard P, et al. Debriefing with good judgment: combining rigorous feedback with genuine inquiry. Anesthesiol Clin 2007;25(2):361–76.

49. Salas E, Klein C, King H, et al. Debriefing medical teams: 12 evidence-based best practices and tips. Jt Comm J Qual Patient Saf 2008;34(9):518–27.

50. Lyndon A, Zlatnik MG, Wachter RM. Effective physician-nurse communication: a patient safety essential for labor and delivery. Am J Obstet Gynecol 2011;205(2): 91–6.

General Anesthesia During the Third Trimester

Any Link to Neurocognitive Outcomes?

Annemaria De Tina, MD, FRCPC[a], Arvind Palanisamy, MD, FRCA[b],*

KEYWORDS

- Fetal neurodevelopment • Fetal surgery
- Developmental neurotoxicity of anesthetics • Maternal anesthesia
- Prenatal exposure • Third trimester anesthesia

KEY POINTS

- Most anesthetic agents have been shown to cause neurotoxicity in the developing rodent and nonhuman primate brain by increasing neuronal apoptosis and inducing long-term behavioral deficits.
- Developmental neurotoxicity of anesthetic agents is well-studied in postnatal rodents, but emerging evidence indicates that this phenomenon also occurs in utero during maternal anesthetic administration in rodents.
- Animal data for third trimester exposure are conflicting although evidence supports the overall notion that prolonged administration of anesthetic agents is detrimental to the fetal brain.
- Emerging evidence suggests that dexmedetomidine does not cause neuroapoptosis, at least in primate models.
- Human studies are sparse and the evidence is conflicting and weak to draw meaningful conclusions or influence current practice.

In the past decade, elegant work from animal studies has conclusively shown that anesthetic agents, both inhalational and intravenous, cause widespread apoptotic neurodegeneration and behavioral abnormalities when administered during critical periods of brain development.[1–4] The most widely evaluated period is the phase of synaptogenesis, which, in humans, extends from late second trimester to the first few years of life.[5,6] Therefore, these preclinical studies have caused a lot of concern

Disclosure Statement: The authors have no disclosures.
[a] Obstetric Anesthesiology, Department of Anesthesiology, Perioperative and Pain Medicine, Brigham and Women's Hospital, 75 Francis Street – CWN L1, Boston, MA 02115, USA;
[b] Department of Anesthesiology, Perioperative and Pain Medicine, Brigham and Women's Hospital, Harvard Medical School, 75 Francis Street – CWN L1, Boston, MA 02115, USA
* Corresponding author.
E-mail address: APALANISAMY@BWH.HARVARD.EDU

Anesthesiology Clin 35 (2017) 69–80
http://dx.doi.org/10.1016/j.anclin.2016.09.007   anesthesiology.theclinics.com

among clinical anesthesiologists.[7] The aim of this review is to elaborate on current preclinical evidence for developmental neurotoxicity of anesthetic agents in animal models and discuss its relevance to humans. Only studies involving anesthesia exposure during mid to late pregnancy are included.

USE OF GENERAL ANESTHESIA DURING THE THIRD TRIMESTER

More than 80,000 parturients undergo nonobstetric surgery in the United States every year.[8] Despite the popularity of neuraxial techniques in obstetric anesthesia, many pregnant women continue to require general anesthesia for either pregnancy-related or nonobstetric surgical procedures during the third trimester.[8–11] These include emergency cesarean deliveries, trauma surgery, surgery for acute surgical conditions such as appendicitis and cholecystitis, and fetal interventions. Although the use of general anesthesia during the third trimester has not been determined precisely, the incidence can be as high as 5% to 44% for cesarean delivery in some European countries.[12,13] Although such high rate of general anesthesia is uncommon in the United States, it is clear that a significant number of pregnant women receive and will continue to receive general anesthesia during the third trimester for a variety of indications in addition to cesarean delivery. Until recently, the neurodevelopmental consequences for the fetus of maternal anesthesia were largely unstudied, despite a solid line of evidence that pharmacologic or environmental influences at this stage of life can cause defective cortical structure and abnormal behavior in adulthood.[14–17] This topic merits further scrutiny for a variety of important reasons. First, most general anesthetic agents are lipophilic, cross the placenta easily, and influence the fetal brain. This is supported by work from Li and colleagues,[18] who confirmed that the fetal brain isoflurane concentration after 6 hours of 1.3% isoflurane administration was comparable to the concentration in the maternal brain (0.40 vs 0.42 μmol/g, respectively). Similarly, propofol crosses the placenta readily,[19] but the overall maternal/fetal ratio of mean plasma propofol concentration was high (5.4 vs 0.35 μg/mL; maternal/fetal ratio of approximately 15),[20] which suggests a more complex pharmacokinetic model. Second, some of the surgical procedures required by pregnant patients may necessitate general anesthesia because of the increased complexity and prolonged duration of surgery. Apart from emergent cesarean deliveries, in most cases, the fetus is a bystander. Third, high concentrations of anesthetic (approximately 1.5 minimal anesthetic concentration) are sometimes required to achieve adequate uterine relaxation and minimize the risk of preterm labor. Thus, clinical necessity may inadvertently increase fetal exposure to general anesthetic agents.

NEURODEVELOPMENTAL EVENTS DURING THE THIRD TRIMESTER

To better understand the impact of neurodevelopmental perturbations during the third trimester, it is essential to sequence the key neurodevelopmental events that unfold during this time period. All neurodevelopmental processes are propelled by a preordained genetic program, which is readily modified by environmental and pharmacologic influences. Neural proliferation and differentiation are essentially complete by late second trimester, and the third trimester is characterized by burgeoning brain connectivity and a 5-fold increase in cerebral cortical volume.[21] Specifically, synapse formation accelerates during this critical period at a rate of 4% every week (approximately 40,000 synapses every minute) and continues at least into the first 2 to 3 years of life. Extensive dendritic arborization, cortical lamination, and myelination overlap with this phase of synaptogenesis. The main drivers of these processes include an array of neurotransmitters, of which γ-amino butyric acid (GABA) and glutamate are critically important.[22–24] Abnormal or unphysiologic stimulation or inhibition of these neurotransmitter systems during this period of early brain circuitry formation, as would occur in the setting of maternal general anesthesia, can have long-standing functional consequences. Fetal exposure to anesthetic agents, which act by modulating GABA and NMDA-subtype of glutamate receptors, therefore, has the potential to disrupt these processes, alter developmental trajectories, and induce circuit malfunction.

PRECLINICAL EVIDENCE FOR GENERAL ANESTHETIC NEUROTOXICITY

Most of our understanding of the developmental neurotoxicity of anesthetic agents derives from preclinical studies in rodents and nonhuman primates. This review focuses specifically on evidence generated from pregnant animal models and applies that knowledge to the framework of clinical obstetric anesthesia to determine the possible implications, if any. All studies are summarized in **Table 1** for easy reference.

Rodent Studies

Historically, the phenomenon of developmental neurotoxicity of anesthetic agents was first reported in neonatal rodents.[1] Ontogenically, the stage of brain development in neonatal rodents (postnatal days 0–7) can be considered equivalent to the human third trimester,[5] and, therefore, the results could be directly applicable to humans. However, this extrapolation ignores the hormonal milieu of pregnancy. Estradiol, progesterone, and oxytocin have all been shown to influence early brain development during pregnancy,[25,26] and particularly during labor and delivery.[27] Considering that this hormonal environment is absent in neonates, it is essential to evaluate only studies in pregnant rodents to draw meaningful conclusions.

Inhalational agents

In one of the earliest studies of its kind, Li and colleagues[18] administered 1.3% isoflurane for 6 hours to rats at embryonic day 21 (E21), a time point that reflects late third trimester. Contrary to findings in neonatal rodents, this well-designed study actually showed a reduction in physiologic apoptosis in the hippocampal CA1 region, without any impairment of either juvenile or adult spatial reference memory and learning in the Morris water maze. Interestingly, when the investigators repeated the experiment with a higher concentration of isoflurane (3% in 100% oxygen for 1 hour),[28] there was evidence of increased apoptosis in the CA1 region of the hippocampus and the retrosplenial cortex, accompanied by an increase in plasma levels of S100beta, an astrocytic protein that is released during early brain injury. Neither control treatment (100% oxygen) nor 1.3% isoflurane for 1 hour were associated with neuroapoptosis. Learning and memory, however, were not evaluated in this study. Consistent with previous findings in rats, a similarly designed study in pregnant guinea pigs failed to show increased neuroapoptosis after administration of an anesthetic "cocktail" of 0.55% isoflurane + 75% N_2O + midazolam 1 mg/kg during the third trimester (gestational day >50, total duration of gestation 59–72 days), although the fetal brains in earlier stages of pregnancy showed remarkable vulnerability to anesthetic-induced damage.[29] When these rodent studies are extended to the late or mid second trimester, there is considerable evidence for the detrimental effects of anesthetic exposure. A single exposure to 1.4% isoflurane (1 minimal anesthetic concentration) for 4 hours during the second trimester (E14) caused long-lasting impairment of spatial working memory and reduced anxiety in the rat offspring.[30] Mechanisms were not explored in this study, but subsequent work has established that mid gestational exposure to inhalational agents such as isoflurane or sevoflurane upregulates the proapoptotic protein caspase-12, downregulates neuroplasticity-associated protein GAP-43, decreases overall synapse numbers in the fetal hippocampus, induces fetal brain inflammation, and increases caspase-3 activation.[31–33] Thus, collectively, it seems that the fetal brain is more vulnerable to the adverse effects of inhalational anesthetic agents during the second rather than the third trimester. This counteracts the prevailing dogma that the best time to perform urgent nonobstetric surgery in pregnancy is during the second trimester, when organogenesis is complete and the risk of preterm labor is low. However, this dogma has never been validated scientifically, and with current evidence that anesthetic agents could be detrimental to early neurodevelopment, it is essential to revisit and challenge this precept.

Intravenous agents

Neurotoxicity data for intravenous anesthetic use during third trimester are not as robust as those for inhalational agents. Intravenous administration of a sedative dose of ketamine for 2 hours in mid pregnancy (E14) caused neuronal loss in the fetal brain, decreased cell proliferation in the hippocampus, induced depression and anxietylike behaviors, and impaired memory during adolescence. These findings were partly related to an imbalance in the expression of NMDA-subtype of glutamate receptors in the hippocampus.[34,35] Furthermore, even a clinically relevant dose of 2 mg/kg ketamine administered to pregnant rats at E17 (early third trimester) decreased cell proliferation in the subventricular zone of the fetal rat cortex,[36] suggesting that neurogenesis could be impaired. Administration of a 2-hour intravenous infusion of propofol (0.4 mg/kg/min) to rats at E18 (third trimester) induced cleaved caspase-3 activation in the fetal brain at 6 hours, and decreased subsequent hippocampal neuronal density at postnatal days 10 and 28. In addition, propofol-exposed offspring demonstrated less exploratory activity in the open field test and impaired spatial working memory in the radial arm maze task.[37] In a separate experiment, the same group also showed that fetal exposure to 2 hours of propofol during the third trimester was associated with poor development of neurologic reflexes in the neonatal period.[38] Collectively, it seems that ketamine and propofol, unlike inhalational agents, consistently cause adverse neurodevelopmental effects when administered during the third trimester. The reasons for this discrepancy, thus far, remain unknown.

Nonhuman Primate Studies

Inhalational and intravenous agents

Ketamine is among the most extensively studied anesthetic agents in nonhuman primate studies. The first study to specifically address the question of fetal neurotoxicity of anesthetic agents was by Slikker and colleagues[39] Here, the investigators administered a 24 hours infusion of ketamine infusion to pregnant macaques during late second trimester (gestational day 122, duration of gestation approximately 165 days) and reported that such exposure was associated with a significant increase in apoptotic neuronal death in the fetal brain compared with control treatment. Although a 24-hour duration of anesthesia is uncommon, if not unlikely, in routine anesthetic practice, these findings have also been reported after a 5 hours anesthetic exposure in utero. Most of the work in this regard comes from Brambrink and colleagues. In a series of experiments in pregnant macaques, Brambrink's work has revealed unique patterns of fetal brain neurodegeneration for commonly administered anesthetic agents. In an experimental paradigm similar to that of Brambrink and colleagues,[40] investigators administered a 10 mg/kg bolus of ketamine followed by an infusion 10 to 85 mg/kg/h to maintain moderate anesthetic depth for 5 hours in pregnant macaques at gestational day 120 (comparable with the human third trimester). The control group received intravenous saline. The animals were monitored extensively; physiologic monitoring

Table 1
Summary of developmental anesthetic neurotoxicity studies in mid-to-late gestation (in alphabetical order)

Author	Drug	Duration	Model	Timing	Trimester	Histopathology	Brain Region Studied	Behavioral Outcome	Results
Brambrink et al,[40] 2012	Ketamine	5 h IV INF	Macaque	E120	Late second	AC3	Multiple brain regions including forebrain, midbrain, cerebellum, and brain stem	None	5-fold increase in apoptosis
Chien et al,[45] 2015	GA for CD	NA	Human	E20–42 wk	Second and third	NA	NA	Autism	Neonates delivered via CD with GA had 52% higher risk of autism compared with vaginal delivery. No significant risk if CD with regional.
Creagh et al,[46] 2015	GA in utero or first 2 y of life	NA	Human	E0 – 2 y	All	NA	NA	Autism	No evidence for association
Creeley et al,[42] 2013	Propofol	5 h IV INF	Macaque	E120	Late second	AC3, silver, fractin, MBP, GFAP, Iba1, PDGFRα, NeuN, DAPI	Multiple brain regions including forebrain, midbrain, cerebellum, and brain stem	None	2.5-fold increase in both apoptotic neurons and oligodendrocytes in the fetal brain.
Creeley et al,[41] 2014	Isoflurane	5 h	Macaque	E120	Late second	AC3, silver, fractin, MBP, GFAP, Iba1, PDGFRα, CC-1, NeuN, DAPI	Multiple brain regions including forebrain, midbrain, cerebellum, and brain stem	None	4-fold increase in neuronal cell death. Oligoapoptosis more severe than neuronal apoptosis.

(continued on next page)

Table 1
(continued)

Author	Drug	Duration	Model	Timing	Trimester	Histopathology	Brain Region Studied	Behavioral Outcome	Results
Dong et al,[36] 2016	Ketamine	Single IP dose	Rat	E17	Third	BrdU and DAPI	Cortex (ventricular zone and subventricular zone)	None	Doses of ketamine 20 mg/kg or greater demonstrated an inhibition of neural cell proliferation in a dose-dependent manner
Kong et al,[32] 2012	1.3% isoflurane	4 h	Rat	E14 - term	Second to third trimester	CHOP, C12a, synapse structure change	Hippocampus	Postnatal spatial memory and learning impairments	Neuronal apoptosis, change in synapse structure.
Kong et al,[31] 2011	1.3% or 3% isoflurane in 30% O$_2$	1 h	Rat	E14	Second	AC3	Hippocampus - C1 region	Postnatal spatial memory and learning impairments in 3% group	3% isoflurane had more neurodegeneration compared with controls and 1.3% isoflurane
Koo et al,[43] 2014	Dexmedetomidine, ketamine	12 h INF	Cynomolgus	E120	Late second	AC3, TUNEL, silver, HE	Frontal cortex, midbrain, cerebellum, medulla and brainstem	None	Dexmedetomidine at low and high doses did not induce apoptosis. Ketamine caused apoptosis and degeneration
Li et al,[38] 2014	Propofol, intralipid	1 vs 2 h vs intralipid 2 vs saline 2 h	Rat	E18	Third	None	None	Slower eye maturation, slower and delayed reflexes	Brain and body weights in 2H propofol group on P10 were lower (no different at P0 or P28).
Li et al,[18] 2007	1.3% isoflurane	6 h	Rat	E21	Third	AC3, TUNEL	Hippocampus, cortex	No memory/learning impairment	Apoptosis decreased at 2 h, but not at 18 h, or postnatal day 5
Palanisamy et al,[30] 2011	1.4% isoflurane	4 h	Rat	E14	Second	None	None	Impaired spatial memory acquisition and reduced anxiety	Deficits in spatial memory after in utero isoflurane exposure

Study	Agent	Duration	Animal	Age	Trimester	Markers	Regions	Behavior	Findings
Rizzi et al,[29] 2008	Isoflurane + N20 + midazolam	4 h	Guinea pig	E50+	Third	AC3, C9, NeuN and Nissl	Retrosplenial, parietal, cingulate, occipital and piriform cortical regions; amygdala, subiculum, hippocampus and anterior thalamus	None	No significant increase in neuroapoptosis in fetus' exposed to anesthesia in the third trimester, but fetal brains in earlier stages of pregnancy showed remarkable vulnerability to anesthetic-induced damage
Slikker et al,[39] 2007	Ketamine	24 h INF	Macaque	E122	Late second	AC3, Fluoro-Jade C, silver, TUNEL, in situ hybridization and autoradiographs, EM	Whole brain	None	Increase in apoptosis. EM findings indicate ketamine cell death is apoptotic and necrotic in nature
Sprung et al,[44] 2009	GA during CD	—	Human	CD	Third	None	None	None	Risk similar in SVD and CD, but reduced in children getting RA + CD then SVD
Wang et al,[28] 2009	1.3 or 3% isoflurane	1 h	Rat	E21	Third	AC3, S100 B in fetal blood	CA1 region of hippocampus and retrosplenial cortex	None	Neurodegeneration in hippocampal and retrosplenial cortex after 1 h of 3%, not 1.3%
Xiong et al,[37] 2014	Propofol, intralipid	2 h	Rat	E18	Third	AC3, synaptophysin, Nissl, NeuN	Hippocampus CA1 and CA3 regions	Exploratory and learning behaviors reduced in propofol group	Increased levels of AC3, neuronal density reduced, synaptophysin levels reduced

(continued on next page)

Table 1
(continued)

Author	Drug	Duration	Model	Timing	Trimester	Histopathology	Brain Region Studied	Behavioral Outcome	Results
Zhao et al,[34] 2014	Ketamine	2 h	Rat	E14	Second	Nissl, BrdU, Golgi-Cox, BDNF, PSD-95, NR1, NR2A, NR2B	Dorsal hippocampus CA1 and CA3 regions	Depression and anxietylike behaviors and impaired memory	Fetal brain exposed to ketamine exhibited neuronal loss, pyramidal neuron abnormalities, and reduced cell proliferation in the hippocampus.
Zhao et al,[35] 2016	Ketamine	2 h	Rat	E14	Second	PSD-95, synaptophysin, NR2A, NR2B, TUNEL, AC3, Nissl, Golgi-Cox	Prefrontal cortex	None	Fetal ketamine exposure caused neuroapoptosis, cell loss, and impaired neuronal development of the prefrontal cortex
Zheng et al,[33] 2013	2.5% sevoflurane for 2 h or 4.1% sevoflurane for 6 h	2 or 6 h	Mice	E14	Second	Interleukin-6, PSD-95, synaptophysin, AC3, B-actin	Entire cerebral hemisphere	Impaired learning and memory	Induced apoptosis, increased IL-6 levels, and reduced postsynaptic density and synaptophysin levels

Abbreviations: AC3, activated caspase-3, a marker for apoptosis; BDNF, brain-derived neurotrophic factor; BrdU, bromodeoxyuridine, marker for cell in the S-phase; C12a, caspase-12 antibody; C9, caspase-9, a marker for apoptosis; CC-1, marker for mature oligodendrocytes; CD, cesarean delivery; CHOP, C/EBP homologous transcription factor protein; DAPI, 4′, 6-diamidino-2-phenylindole (detects abnormal changes in nuclear chromatin pattern indicative of apoptotic cell death); E, embryonic day; EM, electron microscopy; fractin, breakdown product by caspase mediated proteolysis of actin; GA, general anesthesia; GFAP, glial fibrillary acidic protein, a marker for astrocytes; Golgi-Cox, dendritic length and branch number; HE, hematoxylin and eosin staining; Iba1, ionized calcium-binding adaptor molecule 1, a marker for microglia and macrophages; INF, infusion; IP, intraperitoneal; IV, intravenous; MBP, myelin basic protein, identifies young premyelinating and myelinating differentiated oligodendrocytes; NA, not applicable; NeuN, neuronal nuclei antigen, marker for mature neurons; Nissl, neuronal cell body staining; NR1, NR2A, NR2B, N-methyl-D-aspartate (NMDA) receptor subunits; PDGFRα, platelet-derived growth factor receptor alpha, a marker for OL progenitors; PSD-95, postsynaptic density protein 95; silver, DeOlmos cupric silver method; RA, regional anesthesia; SVD, spontaneous vaginal delivery; TUNEL, terminal deoxynucleotidyl transferase dUTP nick end labeling.

and perianesthetic care was comparable with operating room standards. Neuronal death in the fetal brain was assessed 3 hours after cessation of treatment using activated caspase-3, a marker for apoptosis. Ketamine administration was associated with an approximately 5-fold increase in apoptosis in the fetal brain compared with control treatment. The most affected regions of the brain included the cerebellum, caudate nucleus, putamen and nucleus accumbens, a pattern of neurodegeneration that is unique in that the hippocampus, the focus of most rodent studies, was relatively spared.

These studies have since been extended to the more clinically relevant inhalational and intravenous anesthetics. Creeley and colleagues[41] administered 1% to 1.5% isoflurane to maintain moderate surgical plane of anesthesia in late second trimester pregnant macaques (control group animals were handled similarly but did not receive any anesthetic). Similar to ketamine, in utero exposure to isoflurane caused a 4-fold increase in neuronal cell death in the fetal brain compared with control treatment. An interesting aspect of this study was that the investigators also quantified oligodendrocytic cell death after in utero isoflurane exposure, and confirmed that oligoapoptosis was more severe than neuronal apoptosis (59% vs 41% of all apoptotic profiles, respectively). Finally, in a similar study, pregnant rhesus macaques were exposed to 5 hours of either propofol anesthesia or control treatment ("no anesthesia").[42] Animals that received propofol underwent a stable, well-monitored, clinically realistic, and uneventful anesthesia. Three hours later, there was an approximately 2.5-fold increase in both apoptotic neurons and oligodendrocytes in the fetal brains of propofol-treated macaques. Of note, the brain regions most affected by propofol were similar to those affected by isoflurane. Finally, promising recent data suggest that even a 12 hours infusion of high-dose dexmedetomidine in gestational day 120 (second trimester) cynomolgus monkeys had no effect on neuroapoptosis in the frontal cortical layers of the fetal brain.[43] This is not surprising, considering that most adverse neurodevelopmental events have been attributed to modulation of either glutamate or GABA-ergic pathways and not adrenoceptor mechanisms.

With this robust line of evidence from nonhuman primate models, it is clear that the fetal brain is susceptible to maternally administered anesthetic agents in the third trimester, especially when administered for a prolonged period (≥5 h). However, it is not known if a shorter duration of anesthetic administration, which is most often the case in clinical practice, induces similar adverse neuropathologic effects. Furthermore, the 2.5- to 5-fold increase in neuronal apoptosis is modest when compared with rodent studies, but we do not know if such neurodegeneration induces any long-term learning and memory dysfunction. This critical question will only be addressed when shorter durations of anesthetic administration are investigated specifically, along with comprehensive assessment of learning and memory in nonhuman primates.

Population Studies

The relatively robust animal data, however, are not supported by a wealth of human studies. In the only well-designed population-based birth cohort study (Olmsted County, Minnesota),[44] the authors asked the question if exposure to general or regional anesthesia during cesarean delivery increased the risk of learning disabilities in the offspring. Using educational and medical records of all children born between the years 1976 and 1982 in Olmsted County, Minnesota, the authors directly compared the rates of learning disability in offspring who underwent cesarean birth under either general (n = 193) or regional anesthesia (n = 304) and uncomplicated vaginal delivery. The rates of learning disability were no different between the general anesthesia group for cesarean delivery and vaginal birth, but were significantly reduced for babies born after regional anesthesia for cesarean delivery. It is reassuring that even the children whose mothers required emergency general anesthesia (presumably secondary to presumed fetal compromise) did not have an higher incidence of learning disability. However, learning disability is only 1 component of altered brain function and it remains to be seen if other domains of human function are affected. Recent studies have explored the association between general anesthesia during the third trimester and autism spectrum disorders in the offspring, but the results are conflicting. Using a propensity score–matched technique to adjust for underlying risk factors, Chien and colleagues[45] evaluated the link between general anesthesia during cesarean delivery and autism risk in a population-based data set derived from national registries in Taiwan. General anesthesia for cesarean delivery, but not regional anesthesia, was associated with a 52% higher risk for developing autism than vaginal delivery in this study. By contrast, a population-based sibling cohort study from Puerto Rico found no evidence for an association though this study included anesthesia exposures during both pregnancy and during the first 2 years of life.[46] Future studies are required to determine the impact of anesthesia for nonobstetric surgeries and neonatal neurodevelopmental outcomes.

SUMMARY

The third trimester fetal brain seems vulnerable to both inhalational and intravenous anesthetics administered during the third trimester in rodents and nonhuman primates especially when administered for prolonged periods. Most intravenous anesthetic agents investigated, with the exception of dexmedetomidine, consistently produce adverse neurodevelopmental consequences, but the evidence is mixed for inhalational agents. Human studies are unequivocal; general anesthesia during emergent cesarean delivery is not associated with learning disability, but shows a possible association with an increased risk of autism diagnosis. The prevalence of numerous confounding variables, including factors that drive the need for general anesthesia, precludes making a robust determination.

REFERENCES

1. Jevtovic-Todorovic V, Hartman RE, Izumi Y, et al. Early exposure to common anesthetic agents causes widespread neurodegeneration in the developing rat brain and persistent learning deficits. J Neurosci 2003;23(3):876–82.
2. Fredriksson A, Ponten E, Gordh T, et al. Neonatal exposure to a combination of N-methyl-D-aspartate and gamma-aminobutyric acid type A receptor anesthetic agents potentiates apoptotic neurodegeneration and persistent behavioral deficits. Anesthesiology 2007;107(3):427–36.
3. Paule MG, Li M, Allen RR, et al. Ketamine anesthesia during the first week of life can cause long-lasting cognitive deficits in rhesus monkeys. Neurotoxicol Teratol 2011;33(2):220–30.
4. Stratmann G, Sall JW, May LD, et al. Isoflurane differentially affects neurogenesis and long-term neurocognitive function in 60-day-old and 7-day-old rats. Anesthesiology 2009;110(4):834–48.
5. Clancy B, Darlington RB, Finlay BL. Translating developmental time across mammalian species. Neuroscience 2001;105(1):7–17.
6. Dobbing J, Sands J. Comparative aspects of the brain growth spurt. Early Hum Dev 1979;3(1):79–83.

7. Palanisamy A. Maternal anesthesia and fetal neurodevelopment. Int J Obstet Anesth 2012;21(2):152–62.
8. Cheek TG, Baird E. Anesthesia for nonobstetric surgery: maternal and fetal considerations. Clin Obstet Gynecol 2009;52(4):535–45.
9. Goodman S. Anesthesia for nonobstetric surgery in the pregnant patient. Semin Perinatol 2002;26(2):136–45.
10. Jancelewicz T, Harrison MR. A history of fetal surgery. Clin Perinatol 2009;36(2): 227–36, vii.
11. Tran KM. Anesthesia for fetal surgery. Semin Fetal Neonatal Med 2010;15(1): 40–5.
12. Stourac P, Blaha J, Klozova R, et al. Anesthesia for cesarean delivery in the Czech Republic: a 2011 national survey. Anesth Analg 2015;120(6):1303–8.
13. Jenkins JG, Khan MM. Anaesthesia for Caesarean section: a survey in a UK region from 1992 to 2002. Anaesthesia 2003;58(11):1114–8.
14. Berman RF, Hannigan JH. Effects of prenatal alcohol exposure on the hippocampus: spatial behavior, electrophysiology, and neuroanatomy. Hippocampus 2000; 10(1):94–110.
15. Cuzon VC, Yeh PW, Yanagawa Y, et al. Ethanol consumption during early pregnancy alters the disposition of tangentially migrating GABAergic interneurons in the fetal cortex. J Neurosci 2008;28(8):1854–64.
16. Uban KA, Sliwowska JH, Lieblich S, et al. Prenatal alcohol exposure reduces the proportion of newly produced neurons and glia in the dentate gyrus of the hippocampus in female rats. Horm Behav 2010;58(5):835–43.
17. Ang ES Jr, Gluncic V, Duque A, et al. Prenatal exposure to ultrasound waves impacts neuronal migration in mice. Proc Natl Acad Sci U S A 2006;103(34): 12903–10.
18. Li Y, Liang G, Wang S, et al. Effects of fetal exposure to isoflurane on postnatal memory and learning in rats. Neuropharmacology 2007;53(8):942–50.
19. Dailland P, Cockshott ID, Lirzin JD, et al. Intravenous propofol during cesarean section: placental transfer, concentrations in breast milk, and neonatal effects. A preliminary study. Anesthesiology 1989;71(6):827–34.
20. Ngamprasertwong P, Dong M, Niu J, et al. Propofol Pharmacokinetics and estimation of fetal propofol exposure during mid-gestational fetal surgery: a maternal-fetal sheep model. PLoS One 2016;11(1):e0146563.
21. de Graaf-Peters VB, Hadders-Algra M. Ontogeny of the human central nervous system: what is happening when? Early Hum Dev 2006;82(4):257–66.
22. Ben-Ari Y. Excitatory actions of gaba during development: the nature of the nurture. Nat Rev Neurosci 2002;3(9):728–39.
23. Wang DD, Kriegstein AR. Defining the role of GABA in cortical development. J Physiol 2009;587(Pt 9):1873–9.
24. LoTurco JJ, Owens DF, Heath MJ, et al. GABA and glutamate depolarize cortical progenitor cells and inhibit DNA synthesis. Neuron 1995;15(6):1287–98.
25. McCarthy MM. Estradiol and the developing brain. Physiol Rev 2008;88(1): 91–124.
26. Tsutsui K. Progesterone biosynthesis and action in the developing neuron. Endocrinology 2008;149(6):2757–61.
27. Tyzio R, Cossart R, Khalilov I, et al. Maternal oxytocin triggers a transient inhibitory switch in GABA signaling in the fetal brain during delivery. Science 2006; 314(5806):1788–92.
28. Wang S, Peretich K, Zhao Y, et al. Anesthesia-induced neurodegeneration in fetal rat brains. Pediatr Res 2009;66(4):435–40.

29. Rizzi S, Carter LB, Ori C, et al. Clinical anesthesia causes permanent damage to the fetal guinea pig brain. Brain Pathol 2008;18(2):198–210.

30. Palanisamy A, Baxter MG, Keel PK, et al. Rats exposed to isoflurane in utero during early gestation are behaviorally abnormal as adults. Anesthesiology 2011; 114(3):521–8.

31. Kong F, Xu L, He D, et al. Effects of gestational isoflurane exposure on postnatal memory and learning in rats. Eur J Pharmacol 2011;670(1):168–74.

32. Kong FJ, Tang YW, Lou AF, et al. Effects of isoflurane exposure during pregnancy on postnatal memory and learning in offspring rats. Mol Biol Rep 2012;39(4): 4849–55.

33. Zheng H, Dong Y, Xu Z, et al. Sevoflurane anesthesia in pregnant mice induces neurotoxicity in fetal and offspring mice. Anesthesiology 2013;118(3):516–26.

34. Zhao T, Li Y, Wei W, et al. Ketamine administered to pregnant rats in the second trimester causes long-lasting behavioral disorders in offspring. Neurobiol Dis 2014;68:145–55.

35. Zhao T, Li C, Wei W, et al. Prenatal ketamine exposure causes abnormal development of prefrontal cortex in rat. Sci Rep 2016;6:26865.

36. Dong C, Rovnaghi CR, Anand KJ. Ketamine exposure during embryogenesis inhibits cellular proliferation in rat fetal cortical neurogenic regions. Acta Anaesthesiol Scand 2016;60(5):579–87.

37. Xiong M, Li J, Alhashem HM, et al. Propofol exposure in pregnant rats induces neurotoxicity and persistent learning deficit in the offspring. Brain Sci 2014; 4(2):356–75.

38. Li J, Xiong M, Alhashem HM, et al. Effects of prenatal propofol exposure on postnatal development in rats. Neurotoxicol Teratol 2014;43:51–8.

39. Slikker W Jr, Zou X, Hotchkiss CE, et al. Ketamine-induced neuronal cell death in the perinatal rhesus monkey. Toxicol Sci 2007;98(1):145–58.

40. Brambrink AM, Evers AS, Avidan MS, et al. Ketamine-induced neuroapoptosis in the fetal and neonatal rhesus macaque brain. Anesthesiology 2012;116(2): 372–84.

41. Creeley CE, Dikranian KT, Dissen GA, et al. Isoflurane-induced apoptosis of neurons and oligodendrocytes in the fetal rhesus macaque brain. Anesthesiology 2014;120(3):626–38.

42. Creeley C, Dikranian K, Dissen G, et al. Propofol-induced apoptosis of neurones and oligodendrocytes in fetal and neonatal rhesus macaque brain. Br J Anaesth 2013;110(Suppl 1):i29–38.

43. Koo E, Oshodi T, Meschter C, et al. Neurotoxic effects of dexmedetomidine in fetal cynomolgus monkey brains. J Toxicol Sci 2014;39(2):251–62.

44. Sprung J, Flick RP, Wilder RT, et al. Anesthesia for cesarean delivery and learning disabilities in a population-based birth cohort. Anesthesiology 2009;111(2): 302–10.

45. Chien LN, Lin HC, Shao YH, et al. Risk of autism associated with general anesthesia during cesarean delivery: a population-based birth-cohort analysis. J Autism Dev Disord 2015;45(4):932–42.

46. Creagh O, Torres H, Rivera K, et al. Previous Exposure to Anesthesia and Autism Spectrum Disorder (ASD): A Puerto Rican Population-Based Sibling Cohort Study. Bol Asoc Med P R 2015;107(3):29–37.

Obstetric and Anesthetic Approaches to External Cephalic Version

Stephanie Lim, MD[a], Jennifer Lucero, MD[a,b],*

KEYWORDS

- External cephalic version • Neuraxial anesthesia for version
- Management for breech presentation
- Risks and complications of external cephalic version

KEY POINTS

- Breech position is the most common abnormal presentation and ECV is a relatively safe procedure to ameliorate the term breech position.
- Neuraxial anesthesia has been successfully used to improve the outcomes of ECV (improved maternal pain scores and successful version) and has been shown to be cost-effective by reducing multiple ECV attempts and cost of breech cesarean delivery.
- The American College of Obstetricians and Gynecologists has developed an algorithm for management of breech position both in reducing the rates of cesarean delivery after successful version and an approach to an initial failed ECV attempt.

INTRODUCTION

External cephalic version (ECV) is an elective procedure in which the fetus is rotated from breech to vertex presentation through external manipulation of the maternal abdomen.[1–3] This procedure is performed on breech term pregnancies to increase a woman's chance of having a vaginal birth (**Fig. 1**).

Breech Presentation

Breech presentation is the most common abnormal fetal presentation and it complicates approximately 3% to 4% of all pregnancies.[1] It occurs when the fetal extremities or pelvis become engaged in the maternal pelvic inlet. Breech presentation can be suspected

The authors have no financial disclosures.
[a] Division of Obstetric Anesthesia, Department of Anesthesia & Perioperative Care, University California San Francisco School of Medicine, San Francisco, CA 94143, USA; [b] Department of Obstetrics, Gynecology & Reproductive Sciences, University California San Francisco School of Medicine, San Francisco, CA 94143, USA
* Corresponding author. 513 Parnassus Avenue, Room S455e, San Francisco, CA 94143-0464513.
E-mail address: Jennifer.Lucero@ucsf.edu

Anesthesiology Clin 35 (2017) 81–94
http://dx.doi.org/10.1016/j.anclin.2016.09.008
1932-2275/17/© 2016 Elsevier Inc. All rights reserved.

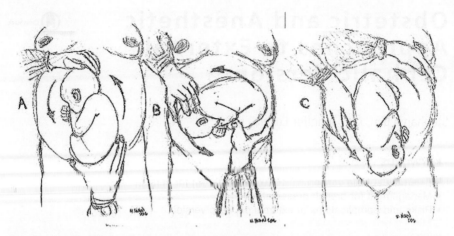

Fig. 1. External cephalic version: fetus is converted from breech to cephalic. (*A*) Forward roll breech is disengaging and simultaneously pushed upward. (*B*) Vertex is simultaneously pushed toward the pelvis. (*C*) Forward roll is completed.

based on clinical examination; however, diagnosis is confirmed with ultrasound. There are 3 types of breech presentations: frank breech, complete breech, and incomplete breech. In frank breech, the fetus's hips are flexed with knees extending bilaterally. In complete breech, both the fetus's hips and knees are flexed. With incomplete breech, either one of fetus's leg or both legs are extended below the buttocks level (**Fig. 2**).

Etiology

Breech presentation likely occurs by chance in most pregnancies. However, in some cases, spontaneous version of the fetus is prevented by maternal anatomic anomalies or fetal anomalies. Normally, the fetus is small in proportion to the amniotic fluid before 28 weeks' gestation and the fetus can rotate to cephalic from breech presentation with ease. As gestational age (GA) and fetal weight increase, the decrease in amniotic fluid volume in relation to the fetus makes the rotation more challenging.

The incidence of singleton breech presentation varies by birth weight and it is inversely related to GA[1] (**Table 1**).

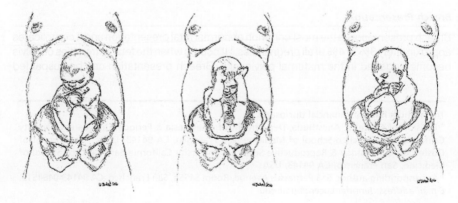

Incomplete breech   Frank breech   Complete Breech

Fig. 2. Types of breech positions.

Table 1 Incidence of singleton breech presentation by birth weight and gestational age		
Birthweight, g	**Gestational Age, wk**	**Incidence, %**
1000	28	35
1000–1499	28–32	25
1500–1999	32–34	20
2000–2499	34–36	8
2500	36	2–3
All weights	—	3–4

Factors Associated with Breech Presentation

There are several maternal and fetal factors associated with breech presentation.[4] Maternal factors include uterine distention from multiparity, previous breech presentation, and abnormal uterine shape (tumors, myoma, pelvic contracture, Müllerian anomalies: septate/bicornate uterus).[4] Fetal conditions associated with breech presentations include short umbilical cord, fetal female gender, hydrocephalus, fetal asphyxia, congenital hip dislocation, anencephalies, spina bifida, meningomyelocele, familial dysautonomia, and chromosomal trisomies (13, 18, and 21).[5] Other obstetric factors may include previous breech delivery, placenta previa or cornual-fundal placenta, extremes of amniotic fluid volume (oligohydramnios and polyhydramnios), and fetal growth restriction.

Management of Breech Presentation

If breech presentation persists beyond GA of 36 weeks, a few strategies should be used and planned for delivery:

- ECV before the onset of labor with a trial of labor if version is successful and cesarean delivery, if version is not successful.
- ECV before the onset of labor with a trial of labor, if version is successful.
- Scheduled cesarean delivery without a trial of ECV.
- A trial of vaginal breech labor for patients who are at low risk of complications from breech delivery.

VAGINAL BREECH DELIVERY

Many maternal and neonatal risks are associated with vaginal breech delivery. The American College of Obstetricians and Gynecologists (ACOG) recommended that the decision regarding vaginal breech delivery depends on the provider's expertise, patient risk factors, and hospital-specific protocols.[6] Informed consent regarding all the serious neonatal and maternal complications should be well documented. Women who are candidates for breech delivery include the following: no placental or cord anomalies, no prior cesarean deliveries, absence of a fetal anomaly that may cause dystocia, estimated fetal weight greater than 2000 g or less than 4000 g, GA ≥36 weeks, absence of fetal head hyperextension, frank or complete beech presentation, spontaneous labor and immediate availability of staff who are skilled in breech delivery, and facilities with capabilities to perform emergency cesarean delivery.

Complications from Vaginal Breech Delivery

The risks associated with vaginal breech delivery include neonatal morbidity, such as intrapartum fetal death, intrapartum fetal asphyxia, cord prolapse, birth trauma, dystocia of head/head entrapment, ischemic encephalopathy, spinal cord injuries, and fetal heart rate abnormalities.[7] ACOG issued an updated committee opinion in 2006 regarding the mode of term singleton breech delivery. The initial committee opinion from ACOG in 2001, based largely from the Term Breech Trial, recommended that planned vaginal delivery of a term singleton breech was no longer appropriate. ACOG cited the increased pooled perinatal and neonatal mortality rates in the vaginal breech group compared with the planned cesarean delivery group. However, since 2001 several publications emerged from the same researchers (Term Breech Trial) in 3 follow-up studies examining both maternal and neonatal outcomes at 3 months and at 2 years postpartum. The investigators found no difference between the cesarean and vaginal delivery groups on both maternal and neonatal outcomes at these time intervals. Several additional retrospective reports from the Netherlands found no increased neonatal morbidity and mortality with vaginal breech deliveries at centers in which there are experienced providers in vaginal breech delivery and adherence to strict protocols for determination of vaginal breech candidates. After review of the literature in 2006, ACOG adjusted their committee opinion to allow for vaginal breech delivery at centers in which there are skilled providers in vaginal breech deliveries, and strict protocols for eligibility and labor management are established and followed. Additionally, ACOG specified that obstetricians should offer and perform ECV, and extensively counsel the woman regarding the possibility of higher perinatal and neonatal morbidity and mortality with vaginal breech delivery compared with a planned cesarean delivery.[6] A recent retrospective observational study from Finland found the incidence of severe neonatal morbidity was 1.3%, which was similar to the rate in the planned cesarean delivery group in the Term Breech Trial published in 2000.[8] Given the limited availability of obstetric providers trained in singleton vaginal breech delivery, the vast majority of term pregnancies with breech presentation are managed with ECV and/or cesarean delivery.

EXTERNAL CEPHALIC VERSION

ECV is the maneuver in which a practitioner externally manipulates the fetus through the abdominal wall to the cephalic position. Another rarely done maneuver called internal podalic version can assist toward breech delivery.

History of External Cephalic Version

ECV has been practiced since the time of Aristotle (384–322 BC).[9] ECVs were performed before term in the mid-1970s because of the belief that the procedure would rarely be successful at term. ECV fell out of favor partly because of perinatal mortality associated with the procedure and the belief that cesarean delivery was a safer option. However, the return of the ECV occurred in the United States in the early 1980s after several studies had favorable results. Many institutions in the United States now offer ECV, as ACOG committee opinion recommends offering ECV and more natural childbirth experiences were desired by mothers.

Procedure/Technique

ECV is performed after obtaining informed consent from the patient and after discussion of risks, benefits, and alternatives. The risks discussed include discomfort/pain during the procedure, possible nausea/vomiting, fetal bradycardia with a potential of prolonged bradycardia resulting in emergency delivery, placental abruption, rupture of membranes, cord prolapse, fetomaternal transfusion, and rarely uterine rupture. An ultrasound examination must be performed to confirm the presentation of the fetus and to rule out fetal or uterine anomalies. A fetal nonstress test must also be performed and the fetal heart tracing must be determined to be reactive. A tocolytic, typically intramuscular (IM) or intravenous (IV) terbutaline, is usually administered to prevent contractions or irritability just before the ECV attempt. Additionally, if the patient is Rh negative, RhoGAM should be administered unless the woman is known to have an Rh-negative fetus or is already sensitized.[10] The technique involves the clinician's hands placed on the patient's abdomen, with one hand lifting the buttocks of the fetus upward and out of the maternal pelvis toward the fundus, while the other hand moves the fetal head toward the maternal pelvis. This technique is called the forward roll.[6] If this attempt is unsuccessful, a backward roll can be tried. During the backward roll, the clinician holds the buttock of the fetus with the left hand, pushes the fetus toward the maternal right flank and upward toward the fundus. The head maybe gently manipulated toward the maternal left flank and downward. At the same time, the clinician applies pressure to the buttock to keep the fetus in a flexed position. In general, steady and slow pressure should be applied on the fetus instead of repeated pushes. Intermittent Doppler tone or ultrasound should be performed to confirm there is no fetal bradycardia. The procedure should be stopped if any sign of fetal distress occurs, multiple attempts are made and unsuccessful, or if anytime the patient is unable to tolerate the procedure. If the version is successful, the patient can be discharged home with instructions and precautions. If unsuccessful, the patient is scheduled for reattempt of ECV at a later date, elective cesarean delivery, or discussion and evaluation of breech vaginal delivery if available at the delivering institution.

Factors Effecting Success of External Cephalic Version

Many prospective and retrospective studies have shown that maternal and neonatal factors influence the success rate of ECV.

Factors associated with lower ECV success rates include the following:[11–13]

- Anterior placenta
- Nulliparity
- Decreased amniotic fluid volume
- Descent of the breech fetus in the pelvis
- Obesity
- Frank breech presentation
- Ruptured membranes
- Abnormally shaped uterus (bicornate)
- Lateral or cornual placenta
- Tense abdominal wall muscle
- Fetal head not palpable
- Thin myometrium

Risks and Contraindications of External Cephalic Version

Complications and risks associated with ECV must be weighed for each individual (**Table 2**). A meta-analysis from 2008 (84 studies, 12,955 women, performed after 36 weeks) showed that serious adverse outcomes were infrequent.[3]

ECV is contraindicated in the settings of increased fetal morbidity or low chance of successful version.[14]

These factors include the following:

- Placenta anomalies that are indicated for cesarean delivery (placenta accreta, placenta previa)
- Fetal or obstetric conditions requiring cesarean delivery

Table 2
Risk of external cephalic version

Outcome	%
Overall complication risk	6.1
Transient fetal heart rate changes	4.7
Fetomaternal transfusion	0.9
Emergency cesarean delivery	0.4
Vaginal bleeding	0.3
Ruptured membranes	0.2
Fetal demise	0.2
Cord prolapse	0.2
Placental abruption	0.2

From Grootscholten K, Kok M, Oei SG, et al. External cephalic version-related risks: a meta-analysis. Obstet Gynecol 2008;112(5):1143–51; with permission.

- Severe oligohydramnios or ruptured membranes
- Nonreassuring fetal heart tones
- Significant fetal or uterine anomaly (hydrocephaly, septate uterus)
- Hyperextended fetal head
- Placental abruption
- Multiple gestations
- Untreated fetal anemia or hydrops

Relative contraindications include maternal hypertension/preeclampsia with severe features, decreased amniotic fluid volume, and fetal growth restriction. In cases of alloimmunization in which the fetus has been treated with intrauterine transfusion and is not anemic, an attempt at ECV is a possibility and up to the discretion of the obstetric provider.

Timing and Outcome

ECV is typically performed near term and if successful the chance the fetus will remain cephalic after ECV is high. When complications during the ECV necessitate urgent cesarean delivery, the term or near-term fetus will likely have fetal lung maturity and will not require prolonged resuscitation. With consensus from major obstetric societies, initial ECVs are usually scheduled at GA ≥37 0/7 weeks in most institutions.[10]

The largest trial is the Early External Cephalic Version 2 Trial, which compared ECV performed at term versus ECV before term.[13] A total of 1543 women with a singleton breech fetus were randomly assigned to ECV at either GA 34 to 36 weeks or at GA ≥37 weeks. The major finding was that early ECV resulted in significantly fewer fetuses in noncephalic presentation at delivery than late ECV (41.1% vs 49.1%; relative risk [RR] 0.84, 95% confidence interval [CI] 0.75–0.94). The rate of cesarean delivery was not significantly reduced with early ECV (52% vs 56%; RR 0.93, 95% CI 0.85–1.02). The early ECV group did not have a significant risk of preterm birth (<37 weeks) when compared with late ECV group (6.5% vs 4.4%, RR 1.48, 95% CI 0.97–2.26). In the trial, the mean GA of both groups at delivery was 39.1 weeks. Each group had a 3% to 4% complication rate with the most common complication being the nonreassuring fetal heart tones.

A Cochrane meta-analysis from 2015 combined 5 trials and concluded that ECV at GA 34 to 36 weeks decreased the rate of noncephalic presentation at delivery (RR

0.81, 95% CI 0.74–0.90) compared with ECV at GA $\geq$37 weeks.[2] However, the analysis failed to show that the decrease in noncephalic presentation did not proportionately result in overall decrease in cesarean delivery rate (RR 0.92, 95% CI 0.85–1.00). Therefore, women should be extensively counseled regarding the advantages and disadvantages of early ECV. The rare complication of delivery of a preterm infant should be weighed against the success of the ECV in the preterm patient. Depending on the individual institution's guidelines and the level of acuity of the neonatal intensive care unit, an early ECV may not be an option.

ANCILLARY MANAGEMENT TO ENHANCE EXTERNAL CEPHALIC VERSION SUCCESS

Many ancillary methods have been tried to improve relaxation of the uterus and maternal abdominal wall muscles to reduce the maternal discomfort/pain of the procedure, allowing for the clinician to manipulate the fetus.

Vibroacoustic Stimulation

One small study investigated the potential role of vibroacoustic stimulation to aid ECV.[15] It is used to stimulate the fetus from its midline spine position to lateral spine position; as a result, manipulating the fetus should be easier and more successful. In one study, 19 of 22 fetuses in the treatment group and 1 of 12 in control group had successful ECV. Larger studies should be performed to determine the efficacy of vibroacoustic stimulation; however, the technique is inexpensive, well tolerated, and has no proven harm.

Moxibustion

Moxibustion, is a traditional Chinese therapy made from *Artemisia argyi* and can be administered directly with an acupuncture needle or burned in close proximity to patient's skin. It has been long believed that when acupuncture with moxibustion is performed at a specific area, such as the outer corner of the toenail (BL67), it helps correct the fetus from a nonvertex to vertex position. A multicenter randomized controlled clinical trial with 406 patients who had ultrasound-confirmed breech pregnancy at GA 33 to 35 weeks were assigned to either true moxibustion, sham moxibustion, or usual care. The primary outcome of the study was to have cephalic presentation at birth: 58.1% of patients from the true moxibustion group were found to have cephalic presentation at term compared with 43.4% in the sham moxibustion group (RR 1.34, 95% CI 1.05–1.70). In the usual care group, 44.8% had cephalic presentation at term (RR 1.29, 95% CI 1.02–1.64). The number needed to treat was found to be 8 (95% CI 4–72) and the authors did not find any severe adverse effects during the treatment.[16] However, there have been more recent single-center randomized controlled clinical trials that have concluded moxibustion did not have any significant effects in correcting breech position.[17,18] Given that there have been no reported adverse effects during the treatment of moxibustion, patients have not been discouraged from using this technique.

Amnioinfusion

Two studies have investigated the efficacy of transabdominal amnioinfusion to help facilitate ECV. In one case series of 6 patients who previously had failed ECV, amnioinfusion with 700–900 mL of warm saline solution resulted in cephalic after repeated ECV.[19] Another cohort study demonstrated that infusion of lactated Ringers solution until an amniotic fluid index of 15 did not improve the ECV success.[20] Both studies had a small number of patients, and also had discordant results. This potential procedure lacks data to support its efficacy, carries potential risk of rupture of amniotic membranes, and chorioamnionitis. Therefore, it is not a recommended approach for ECV.

Tocolysis

Beta-1 agonists, such as terbutaline, ritodrine, and salbutamol, are used as tocolytics agents. Their side effects are maternal and fetal tachycardia and are usually well tolerated. Most institutions offer 1 dose of terbutaline 0.25 mg IM or IV 15 minutes before the ECV procedure. A review from 2015 compiled 6 trials of ECV with or without tocolysis.[2] The conclusion from the review was that tocolysis administration is associated with increased prevalence of cephalic presentation in labor (RR 1.68, 95% CI 1.14–2.48) compared with no tocolytics use and cesarean delivery rate is reduced in both nulliparous and multiparous women (RR 0.77, 95% CI 0.67–0.88).

Nitroglycerin

Nitroglycerin is a rapid and effective uterine muscle relaxant agent. A systematic review from 2002 found that small doses of nitroglycerin administered in various routes (IV, SL, patch) was not effective for relaxing the uterus compared with placebo for preterm contractions, fetal extraction during cesarean delivery, and ECV.[21] Another trial compared sublingual nitroglycerin (0.8 mg) versus IV ritodrine (111 µg/min) given before ECV and found that the nitroglycerin group had more side effects, such as headache and blood pressure changes.[22] Furthermore, patients in the sublingual (SL) nitroglycerin group had fewer successful versions.

Calcium Channel Blockers

Nifedipine, one of many calcium channel blockers, has been used as a tocolytic agent for preterm labor. A review article from 2011 looked at 2 trials that used nifedipine. In 1 of the 2 studies, nifedipine was compared with terbutaline. The other study compared nifedipine with a placebo and both concluded that the use of nifedipine did not increase the prevalence of cephalic presentation in labor, and it did not lower the rate of cesarean delivery.[23]

Analgesia

Many centers do not routinely offer analgesia for ECV. ECV is associated with maternal anxiety, pain, and discomfort. The maternal discomfort during the procedure can often be significant enough that the obstetrician has to prematurely terminate the ECV.

Remifentanil

A randomized, double-blinded, controlled trial with women of GA 36 to 41 weeks with breech presentation either received remifentanil infusion of 0.1 µg/kg per minute with demand bolus of 0.1 µg/kg, or saline as a placebo.[24] A total of 29 patients in the placebo group versus 31 in remifentanil group were enrolled. Women who received remifentanil had significantly reduced pain scores compared with placebo (placebo 6.5 ± 2.4 vs remifentanil 4.7 ± 2.5, $P = .005$). However, the pain scores at 10 minutes were not significantly different between groups ($P = .054$). The success rates of ECV were not different between the 2 groups (remifentanil group 54.8% vs placebo 41.3%, $P = .358$). In addition, the incidence of adverse outcomes was not statistically different between the 2 groups.

Nitrous Oxide

One prospective study compared 150 women with singleton pregnancy and breech presentation at term who underwent ECV with N2O for analgesia (50:50 mix with oxygen), with 150 ECVs with no analgesia.[25] Women who received N2O had a statistically lower level of pain (median, 6; range, 4–7), compared with no analgesia (median, 7; range, 5–8; $P<.01$). No differences in success rate or perinatal outcomes were found.

Remifentanil Versus Nitrous Oxide

Another randomized open-label study evaluated the effect of remifentanil versus nitrous oxide on ECV success.[26] The study enrolled 60 patients in each group, and found the success rate was the same (31/60, 51.7%). Pain scores were significantly lower in the remifentanil group (3.2 ± 2.4 vs 6.0 ± 2.3; $P<.01$). Although the study did not find any differences between the 2 groups for ECV-related complications, there was a higher incidence of adverse effects in the remifentanil group (21.7 events/100 women vs 6.7 events/100 women with nitrous oxide, $P = .03$). The adverse effects were mild, reversible, and predictably related to narcotics.

Neuraxial Analgesia

Many studies have shown that neuraxial analgesia (spinal, epidural, or combined spinal-epidural [CSE]) has increased success rates and improved maternal pain scores. One prospective study compared IV fentanyl versus CSE (intrathecal: bupivacaine plus fentanyl).[27] There was no difference in ECV success rate; however, median visual analog pain scores (0–100 mm scale) were significantly lower in the group that received CSE (3 [0–12]) compared with IV fentanyl (36 [16–54]) ($P<.005$). Patients' satisfaction (0–10 scale) was also higher in the CSE group (10 [9–10]) versus the IV fentanyl group (7 [4–9]) ($P<.005$).

Neuraxial analgesia also provides relaxation to maternal abdominal wall muscles, which could provide additional ease in the external movement of the fetus. Another benefit of having neuraxial anesthesia is the avoidance of general anesthesia and airway management in the event of an emergency cesarean delivery from complications during the ECV attempt.

Several randomized control trials showed that higher success rates of ECV are attributable to neuraxial anesthesia. Six published randomized controlled trials showed that compared with IV analgesia or placebo, neuraxial anesthesia had a higher success rate of ECV (59% vs 37.6%, RR 1.58, CI 1.29–1.93).[28] Neuraxial anesthesia use was associated with an 11% reduction in cesarean delivery rate (59.3% to 48.4%), but this difference was not statistically significant. The number needed to treat to have 1 additional successful ECV was 5 with the use of neuraxial anesthesia.

Neuraxial Anesthesia Dose and Complications

In reviewing published studies, it is apparent that there is a dose response effect of neuraxial anesthesia to ECV success. The dose of neuraxial anesthesia, sample size, and success rates of different studies are listed in **Table 3**.

The higher doses were also associated with more complications, such as maternal hypotension and fetal bradycardia. In some of the studies, the neonates required urgent delivery for sustained fetal bradycardia. At some centers, the ECV is performed in the labor room or triage, in these situations it is important for the anesthesiologist and pediatrician to be readily available in the event of a prolonged or sustained fetal bradycardia.

Table 3
Randomized controlled trials of external cephalic version, neuraxial anesthesia dosing, and external cephalic version success rate

Author, Published Year	Sample Size	Anesthetic Technique and Dose	Treatment Group Success Rate, %	Control Group Success Rate, %	P
Sullivan et al,[27] 2009	95	Combined spinal-epidural, bupivacaine 2.5 mg and fentanyl 15 µg vs intravenous fentanyl 50 µg	47	31	.14
Schorr et al,[29] 1997	69	Epidural, lidocaine 2% with epinephrine 5 µg/mL (up to T6 level) vs no analgesia	69	32	.01
Dugoff et al,[30] 1999	102	Spinal, bupivacaine 2.5 mg, sufentanil 10 µg vs no analgesia	44	42	.863
Mancuso et al,[31] 2000	108	Epidural, lidocaine 2%, fentanyl 100 µg vs no analgesia	59	33	<.05
Weiniger et al,[32] 2007	74	Spinal, bupivacaine 2.5 mg vs no analgesia	67	32	.004
Weiniger et al,[33] 2010	64	Spinal, bupivacaine 7.5 mg vs no analgesia	87	58	.009

Cost-effective Analysis of Neuraxial Anesthesia

One study investigated the cost of neuraxial anesthesia during ECV attempts.[34] The investigators used several published studies on ECV rates and delivery costs to perform a cost-effective analysis. From several published studies the probability of success rate of ECV with neuraxial anesthesia was determined to be 60% compared with an average of 38% without neuraxial anesthesia. Based on the published articles, the investigators estimated the mean delivery costs including ECV with anesthesia equaled $8931 (2.5th–97.5th percentile prediction interval $8541–$9252). If ECV was performed without anesthesia, the cost was $9207 (2.5th–97.5th percentile prediction interval $8896–$9419). The cost discrepancy highlights the increased ECV success with neuraxial anesthesia, both by reducing the multiple attempts at ECV and reduction in breech cesarean delivery.

POSTPROCEDURE
Fetal Monitoring

After the ECV attempt, regardless of success, continuous fetal and external tocometry monitoring is routinely performed. The fetus usually has a transient stress from decreased placental flow during the ECV attempts and the heart rate tracings can be nonreactive for up to 40 minutes.[35]

Anti-D Immune Globulin

One potential risk of ECV is placental abruption and transfusion of fetal blood toward maternal circulation. Women with negative Rh status can be at risk for Rh alloimmunization from ECV attempts. In one prospective observational study, the investigators enrolled patients undergoing ECV with GA ≥36 weeks and did the Kleihauer-Betke test before and after ECVs.[36] In an observational study of 1244 patents with a negative test before ECV, 30 (2.4%) had a positive Kleihauer-Betke test after ECV attempts. Currently, the Kleihauer-Betke test is not recommended. In patients who are Rh- current ACOG guidelines state anti-D immunoglobulin should be administered if delivery of the patient is not anticipated in the next 72 hours.

Management after Successful External Cephalic Version

ACOG currently does not recommend immediate induction after successful ECV. The rate of reversion to breech fetus is very small, and elective induction without onset of labor has been shown to increase neonatal morbidity, increase the risk of cesarean delivery, increase the labor course, and result in greater health care costs.

One recently published study identified the factors associated with cesarean delivery even after successful ECV.[37] This prospective study had 647 women who had a successful uncomplicated ECV. Among 627, 33 (8.5%) of 387 women with spontaneous labor had cesarean delivery versus 59 (24.6%) of 240 who were induced ($P<.001$). Multivariate analysis of those patients showed that higher body mass index ($P = .006$), induction of labor ($P = .001$), and a previous cesarean delivery ($P<.001$)

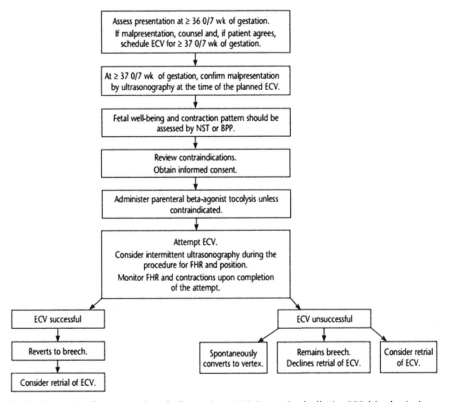

Fig. 3. Algorithm for external cephalic version, ACOG practice bulletin. BPP, biophysical profile; FHR, fetal heart rate; NST, nonstress test. (*From* American College of Obstetricians and Gynecologists' Committee on Practice Bulletins—Obstetrics. Practice Bulletin No. 161: external cephalic version. Obstet Gynecol 2016;127(2):e57–61; with permission.)

were found to be associated with cesarean delivery. Additionally, timing between ECV and delivery was found to be inversely associated with cesarean delivery.

Management after Unsuccessful External Cephalic Version

When the ECV is unsuccessful or the fetus reverts to the breech position, 1 or 2 more attempts can be done in the next few days. Some institutions recommend a second or third attempt of ECV under neuraxial anesthesia and, if unsuccessful, immediate cesarean delivery (**Fig. 3**).

Spontaneous Version

Incidence of spontaneous version to vertex after failed ECV is small. One pooled study showed that spontaneous version to vertex after failed ECV, but before the onset of labor was 0.09% among 210 patients. Multiparous women were found to have higher rate of spontaneous version to vertex compared with nulliparous.[38]

SUMMARY

ECV should be recommended to women with a breech singleton pregnancy if there are no contraindications. ECV increases the chance of cephalic presentation at the onset of labor and decreases the rate of cesarean delivery by almost 40%.[2] The success rate of ECV is approximately 60%; however, maternal, neonatal, and obstetric factors influence the success rate.[3] Beta stimulant tocolysis (eg, terbutaline) improves the success rate of ECV. Neuraxial anesthesia with the beta stimulant tocolysis has been shown to have a higher success rate than tocolytics alone, but with a potential increase in fetal bradycardia. Review of the risks/benefits for the timing of ECV and the number of attempts should be discussed with the patient.

REFERENCES

1. Hickok DE, Gordon DC, Milberg JA, et al. The frequency of breech presentation by gestational age at birth: a large population-based study. Am J Obstet Gynecol 1992;166(3):851–2.
2. Cluver C, Gyte GM, Sinclair M, et al. Interventions for helping to turn term breech babies to head first presentation when using external cephalic version. Cochrane Database Syst Rev 2015;(2):CD000184.
3. Grootscholten K, Kok M, Oei SG, et al. External cephalic version-related risks: a meta-analysis. Obstet Gynecol 2008;112(5):1143–51.
4. Fruscalzo A, Londero AP, Salvador S, et al. New and old predictive factors for breech presentation: our experience in 14 433 singleton pregnancies and a literature review. J Matern Fetal Neonatal Med 2014;27(2):167–72.
5. Moessinger AC, Blanc WA, Marone PA, et al. Umbilical cord length as an index of fetal activity: experimental study and clinical implications. Pediatr Res 1982;16(2):109–12.
6. ACOG Committee on Obstetric Practice. ACOG Committee Opinion No. 340. Mode of term singleton breech delivery. Obstet Gynecol 2006;108(1):235–7.
7. Su M, McLeod L, Ross S, et al. Factors associated with maternal morbidity in the Term Breech Trial. J Obstet Gynaecol Can 2007;29(4):324–30.
8. Macharey G, Ulander VM, Heinonen S, et al. Risk factors and outcomes in "well-selected" vaginal breech deliveries: a retrospective observational study. J Perinat Med 2016. [Epub ahead of print].
9. Coco AS, Silverman SD. External cephalic version. Am Fam Physician 1998;58(3):731–8, 742-734.

10. American College of Obstetricians and Gynecologists' Committee on Practice Bulletins–Obstetrics. Practice Bulletin No. 161: external cephalic version. Obstet Gynecol 2016;127(2):e54–61.

11. Ben-Meir A, Erez Y, Sela HY, et al. Prognostic parameters for successful external cephalic version. J Matern Fetal Neonatal Med 2008;21(9):660–2.

12. Kok M, Cnossen J, Gravendeel L, et al. Clinical factors to predict the outcome of external cephalic version: a metaanalysis. Am J Obstet Gynecol 2008;199(6): 630.e1-7 [discussion: e1–5].

13. Hutton EK, Hannah ME, Ross SJ, et al. The Early External Cephalic Version (ECV) 2 trial: an international multicentre randomised controlled trial of timing of ECV for breech pregnancies. BJOG 2011;118(5):564–77.

14. Rosman AN, Guijt A, Vlemmix F, et al. Contraindications for external cephalic version in breech position at term: a systematic review. Acta Obstet Gynecol Scand 2013;92(2):137–42.

15. Johnson RL, Elliott JP. Fetal acoustic stimulation, an adjunct to external cephalic version: a blinded, randomized crossover study. Am J Obstet Gynecol 1995; 173(5):1369–72.

16. Vas J, Aranda-Regules JM, Modesto M, et al. Using moxibustion in primary healthcare to correct non-vertex presentation: a multicentre randomised controlled trial. Acupunct Med 2013;31(1):31–8.

17. Coulon C, Poleszczuk M, Paty-Montaigne MH, et al. Version of breech fetuses by moxibustion with acupuncture: a randomized controlled trial. Obstet Gynecol 2014;124(1):32–9.

18. Bue L, Lauszus FF. Moxibustion did not have an effect in a randomised clinical trial for version of breech position. Dan Med J 2016;63(2):1–6.

19. Benifla JL, Goffinet F, Bascou V, et al. Transabdominal amnio-infusion facilitates external version maneuver after initial failure. Six successful attempts. J Gynecol Obstet Biol Reprod (Paris) 1995;24(3):319–22 [in French].

20. Adama van Scheltema PN, Feitsma AH, Middeldorp JM, et al. Amnioinfusion to facilitate external cephalic version after initial failure. Obstet Gynecol 2006; 108(3 Pt 1):591–2.

21. Morgan PJ, Kung R, Tarshis J. Nitroglycerin as a uterine relaxant: a systematic review. J Obstet Gynaecol Can 2002;24(5):403–9.

22. Bujold E, Boucher M, Rinfret D, et al. Sublingual nitroglycerin versus placebo as a tocolytic for external cephalic version: a randomized controlled trial in parous women. Am J Obstet Gynecol 2003;189(4):1070–3.

23. Wilcox CB, Nassar N, Roberts CL. Effectiveness of nifedipine tocolysis to facilitate external cephalic version: a systematic review. BJOG 2011;118(4):423–8.

24. Munoz H, Guerra S, Perez-Vaquero P, et al. Remifentanil versus placebo for analgesia during external cephalic version: a randomised clinical trial. Int J Obstet Anesth 2014;23(1):52–7.

25. Burgos J, Cobos P, Rodriguez L, et al. Is external cephalic version at term contraindicated in previous caesarean section? A prospective comparative cohort study. BJOG 2014;121(2):230–5 [discussion: 235].

26. Burgos J, Pijoan JI, Osuna C, et al. Increased pain relief with remifentanil does not improve the success rate of external cephalic version: a randomized controlled trial. Acta Obstet Gynecol Scand 2016;95(5):547–54.

27. Sullivan JT, Grobman WA, Bauchat JR, et al. A randomized controlled trial of the effect of combined spinal-epidural analgesia on the success of external cephalic version for breech presentation. Int J Obstet Anesth 2009;18(4):328–34.

28. Goetzinger KR, Harper LM, Tuuli MG, et al. Effect of regional anesthesia on the success rate of external cephalic version: a systematic review and meta-analysis. Obstet Gynecol 2011;118(5):1137–44.
29. Schorr SJ, Speights SE, Ross EL, et al. A randomized trial of epidural anesthesia to improve external cephalic version success. Am J Obstet Gynecol 1997;177(5): 1133–7.
30. Dugoff L, Stamm CA, Jones OW 3rd, et al. The effect of spinal anesthesia on the success rate of external cephalic version: a randomized trial. Obstet Gynecol 1999;93(3):345–9.
31. Mancuso KM, Yancey MK, Murphy JA, et al. Epidural analgesia for cephalic version: a randomized trial. Obstet Gynecol 2000;95(5):648–51.
32. Weiniger CF, Ginosar Y, Elchalal U, et al. External cephalic version for breech presentation with or without spinal analgesia in nulliparous women at term: a randomized controlled trial. Obstet Gynecol 2007;110(6):1343–50.
33. Weiniger CF, Ginosar Y, Elchalal U, et al. Randomized controlled trial of external cephalic version in term multiparae with or without spinal analgesia. Br J Anaesth 2010;104(5):613–8.
34. Carvalho B, Tan JM, Macario A, et al. Brief report: a cost analysis of neuraxial anesthesia to facilitate external cephalic version for breech fetal presentation. Anesth Analg 2013;117(1):155–9.
35. Hofmeyr GJ, Sonnendecker EW. Cardiotocographic changes after external cephalic version. Br J Obstet Gynaecol 1983;90(10):914–8.
36. Boucher M, Marquette GP, Varin J, et al. Fetomaternal hemorrhage during external cephalic version. Obstet Gynecol 2008;112(1):79–84.
37. Burgos J, Iglesias M, Pijoan JI, et al. Probability of cesarean delivery after successful external cephalic version. Int J Gynaecol Obstet 2015;131(2):192–5.
38. Ben-Meir A, Elram T, Tsafrir A, et al. The incidence of spontaneous version after failed external cephalic version. Am J Obstet Gynecol 2007;196(2):157.e151-3.

Update in the Management of Patients with Preeclampsia

Nerlyne K. Dhariwal, MD, Grant C. Lynde, MD, MBA*

KEYWORDS

- Preeclampsia • Biomarkers • Magnesium sulfate • Hypertension
- Renal dysfunction

KEY POINTS

- Gestational hypertension and preeclampsia develop after 20 weeks' gestation and resolve after delivery of the fetus. Preeclampsia is diagnosed by the presence of hypertension and either proteinuria or signs and symptoms of end-organ dysfunction.
- Risk factors for developing preeclampsia include prior history of preeclampsia, multiple gestation pregnancy, obesity, preexisting hypertension, and preexisting renal disease.
- Monitoring for progression of disease is essential for optimal management of both mother and fetus, with the intent of delivering the fetus as maximally developed as possible while weighing the risks of continuing the pregnancy.

INTRODUCTION

Hypertensive disorders of pregnancy complicate approximately 10% of all deliveries in the United States and is a leading cause of both maternal and fetal morbidity and mortality. Although great efforts have been undertaken to better understand and prevent preeclampsia, little improvement in maternal and fetal outcomes has been observed. Whether a pregnancy is complicated by preexisting hypertension or by preeclampsia, it is essential that a patient's obstetric team monitor the patient's health more frequently to more rapidly identify and treat worsening hypertension. Close monitoring of fetal development is also important to optimally time delivery. This article reviews current knowledge of the factors important to the development of preeclampsia and discusses the anesthetic management of the hypertensive peripartum patient.

The authors have nothing to disclose.
Department of Anesthesiology, Emory University, 1354 Clifton Road Northeast, Atlanta, GA 30322, USA
* Corresponding author.
E-mail address: glynde@emory.edu

Anesthesiology Clin 35 (2017) 95–106
http://dx.doi.org/10.1016/j.anclin.2016.09.009   **anesthesiology.theclinics.com**

DEFINITIONS

Hypertension presenting during pregnancy may be 1 of 4 distinct disease processes:

- Chronic hypertension
- Gestational hypertension
- Preeclampsia
- Chronic hypertension superimposed with preeclampsia

Chronic hypertension is defined as hypertension that exists either before pregnancy or hypertension that develops during pregnancy and fails to resolve by 12 weeks postpartum.[1] Gestational hypertension is defined as an elevation in blood pressure after 20 weeks' gestation without proteinuria or systemic findings. Preeclampsia is defined as hypertension in association with either proteinuria (>300 mg in 24 hours), thrombocytopenia (<100,000/μL), impaired liver function, renal insufficiency (>1.1 mg/dL), pulmonary edema, or new-onset cerebral or visual disturbances.[1,2] Early-onset preeclampsia occurs between 20 weeks' and 34 weeks' gestation. Late-onset preeclampsia develops on, or after, 34 weeks. Table 1 displays characteristics differentiating gestational hypertension from mild and severe preeclampsia.

Although preeclampsia has traditionally been defined as new-onset hypertension and proteinuria, a subset of preeclamptic women presents with hypertension and systemic signs without proteinuria. For this reason, the definition of signs and symptoms defining preeclampsia has broadened to become more inclusive of these patients.[2]

Severe preeclampsia is defined as a systolic blood pressure of 160 mm Hg or greater or a diastolic blood pressure of 110 mm Hg or greater on 2 occasions at least 4 hours apart.[2]

Eclampsia is defined by seizure activity in the presence of preeclampsia. Although it typically presents as a late manifestation after other systemic signs of disease, it can present without other warning signs.

Chronic hypertension superimposed with preeclampsia can present both diagnostic and treatment challenges. This diagnosis is made when a woman with preexisting hypertension after 20 weeks' gestation presents with a sudden exacerbation in hypertension, development of signs or symptoms consistent with preeclampsia

Table 1
Comparison of signs and symptoms of gestational hypertension, mild preeclampsia, and severe preeclampsia

Symptom	Gestational Hypertension	Mild Preeclampsia	Severe Preeclampsia
Systolic blood pressure	140 mm Hg	140 mm Hg	160 mm Hg
Diastolic blood pressure	90 mm Hg	90 mm Hg	110 mm Hg
Proteinuria	None	300 mg/24 h or 1 + Proteinuria on dipstick or Protein/creatinine ratio ≥0.3 mg/dL	≥2 g/24 h or 3 + Proteinuria on a dipstick
Thrombocytopenia	Normal	Normal	<100,000
Liver function tests	Normal	Normal	2× Normal
Creatinine	Normal	Normal	1.1 mg/dL
Pulmonary edema	No	No	Yes
Cerebral disturbances	No	No	Yes
Visual disturbances	No	No	Yes

(proteinuria, increase in liver enzymes, and thrombocytopenia below 100,000/uL), right upper quadrant pain, pulmonary edema, or renal insufficiency. Development of hypertension superimposed with preeclampsia has a worse prognosis for both mother and fetus than either clinical condition alone.

EPIDEMIOLOGY AND RISK FACTORS FOR PREECLAMPSIA

Predicting whether or not a particular pregnancy will be complicated by preeclampsia is important to ensure the mother receives optimal care. Because current science does not have preventive therapies, predicting the risk of preeclampsia should lead to more optimal treatment of the progression of a patient's hypertension as well as reducing the severity of the disease. The incidence of preeclampsia is approximately 3% to 5% of all pregnancies, with a majority of cases presenting with late onset.[3–5] Approximately one-third of all pregnancy-related deaths are due to complications of preeclampsia at a rate of 1.5/100,000 live births. Approximately 40% of these deaths are attributable to cerebrovascular events.[6] Early-onset preeclampsia increases the risk of fetal death (odds ratio = 5.8). Additionally, early-onset preeclampsia is associated with a significantly increased odds ratio for perinatal death and severe neonatal morbidity (odds ratio = 16.4). Although the prognosis for the fetus remains above baseline in late-onset preeclampsia, the odds ratio for perinatal death and severe neonatal morbidity is only 2.0.[3]

Several risk factors have been identified that place women at higher risk for developing preeclampsia during their pregnancy (**Box 1**). Most importantly, a history of preeclampsia in previous pregnancies increases a woman's relative risk by 7.6 times.[7] Multiple gestation pregnancy triples a woman's risk of developing preeclampsia, with the risk increasing even more for triplet versus twin gestation.[8] Preexisting conditions, such as insulin-dependent diabetes, obesity, renal disease, and hypertension, are all associated with an increased risk for developing preeclampsia.[4,9–11] Despite efforts to identify risk factors leading to the development of preeclampsia, at least two-thirds of all affected pregnancies are born to nulliparous women with no other apparent risk factors.[12]

PATHOGENESIS

Failure of embryonic trophoblasts to adequately invade the uterus and spiral arteries, transforming them into low-resistance vessels, marks the beginning of the process

---

Box 1
Risk factors for developing preeclampsia

Age $\geq$40 y

Chronic autoimmune disease

Family history

Type 1 diabetes mellitus

Multiple gestation

Nulliparity

Obesity

Preexisting hypertension

Preexisting renal disease

Previous preeclampsia

that ultimately develops into preeclampsia. Trophoblast cells are the first cells that differentiate from the fertilized egg and ultimately allow implantation of the embryo to implant in the uterus. These cells ultimately form the outer membrane of the placenta and are responsible for the exchange of nutrients and oxygen between mother and fetus. By week 10, the trophoblastic invasion leads to apoptosis of the muscularis layer of the spiral arteries, resulting in a low-pressure vascular bed.[13] Although the exact mechanism by which the muscularis layer undergoes remodeling, it is currently believed that trophoblast cells interact with maternal uterine natural killer (uNK) cells.[14] Decreased, or absent, trophoblast cells due to inflammatory processes or uNK cells lead to failed spiral artery remodeling – ultimately resulting in a high-flow/high-pressure state.[14,15] As opposed to a normal pregnancy, the myometrium of the preeclamptic patient remains responsive to endogenous and exogenous adrenergic stimuli.[16,17]

The high-pressure/high-flow state that exists in the preeclamptic spiral arteries results in sheer stress of the endothelium. Additionally, the forming placenta is at risk for ischemia-reperfusion injury due to spontaneous vasoconstriction of maternal arteries.[15] These injuries lead to the rapid generation of reactive oxygen radicals, resulting in further endothelial injury.[18]

Several circulating factors released by injured endothelial cells cause distal endothelial injury and dysfunction, accounting for the systemic effects seen in severe preeclampsia.[19,20] Some of these factors are in the class of antiangiogenic proteins, which include fms-like tyrosine kinase 1 (sFLT-1). sFLT-1 binds vascular endothelial growth factor (VEGF), preventing VEGF signaling, which ultimately results in hypertension, proteinuria, and glomerular endotheliosis.[21,22]

Another antiangiogenic protein that has been identified as possibly involved with the pathogenesis of preeclampsia is endoglin. Endoglin is a glycoprotein located on cell surfaces and is a transforming growth factor β receptor coreceptor that interacts with sFLT-1 and may result in preeclampsia. Elevated levels of endoglin have been seen in women who subsequently develop preeclampsia.[23] Further research into the roles of endoglin and sFLT-1 are currently in progress with the anticipation of both predicting at-risk pregnancies and possible therapies.

PREVENTION

No effective therapy has been developed to consistently prevent the development of preeclampsia. This is most likely because the disease's pathogenesis occurs weeks before the patient becomes symptomatic. Most therapies aim to reduce the effects of the inflammatory cascade that is manifest in later disease.

Low-dose aspirin has been proposed to reduce the incidence of preeclampsia. Endothelial dysfunction and resultant platelet and clotting system activation are believed to be significant components of the symptoms seen later in preeclampsia. Through its ability to block thromboxane generation, aspirin is thought to reduce the frequency and severity of preeclampsia.

Several smaller trials revealed mixed results; however, the Cochrane Database of Systematic Reviews performed a meta-analysis of 59 trials, including 37,560 women and found a 17% reduction in the development of preeclampsia when women at risk take a low-dose aspirin with a reassuring safety profile.[24] The American College of Obstetricians and Gynecologists Task Force on Hypertension in Pregnancy[2] suggests initiating daily low-dose aspirin beginning in the late first trimester for women with chronic hypertension or with either 2 prior pregnancies complicated by preeclampsia or with 1 pregnancy complicated by preeclampsia and preterm delivery.

Other interventions, including supplementation with vitamins C and E, have been suggested to reduce the oxidative stress seen in preeclamptic patients. These trials as well as a meta-analysis by the *Cochrane Database of Systematic Reviews* have failed to demonstrate benefit.[25,26] Supplementation with other nutritional supplements, such as vitamin D, oral magnesium, and calcium, have demonstrated no benefit in reducing the incidence or severity of preeclampsia either.[27–29]

MANAGEMENT

Management of preeclamptic patients is focused on balancing the risks to both mother and fetus of continuing the pregnancy with the benefits to the fetus of delivering it as fully developed as possible. Current recommendations are to deliver women who present with severe preeclampsia at or beyond 37 0/7 weeks of gestation. Additionally, women between 34 0/7 and 37 0/7 weeks with progressive labor, rupture of membranes, intrauterine growth retardation, oligohydramnios, or a biophysical profile of 6/10 or less should also be delivered. Finally, delivery should occur immediately in suspected cases of fetal abruption.[2]

Monitoring

Current guidelines recommend close monitoring of the hypertensive gravid patient. Daily checks of fetal movement, including kick counts, should be performed by the mother. Additionally, the mother should perform daily self-assessment and report severe headaches, visual changes, epigastric pain, and shortness of breath. Additionally, she should seek assistance if she persistently experiences these symptoms or signs of labor, rupture of membranes, decreased fetal movement, or abruption.

Blood pressure should be checked twice a week and can be performed by the patient or her physicians. Additionally, weekly urine protein analysis should be performed by the patient's health care providers to identify onset and worsening of preeclampsia. In preeclamptic patients, weekly liver enzymes and serum creatinine levels should also be measured. Weekly ultrasound measurements of amniotic fluid volume should be performed. Nonstress tests should be performed weekly in patients with gestational hypertension and twice a week in patients who have mild preeclampsia.

Medications (Antihypertensives)

The goal of antihypertensive therapy is to prevent severe gestational hypertension and reduce the risk of maternal hemorrhagic stroke. The use of antihypertensives in patients who present with mild hypertension seems to reduce the rate of progression to severe hypertension in half but does not affect the incidence of developing preeclampsia.[30] The risk of administering antihypertensives is that it increases the incidence of small-for-gestational-age infants. Current recommendations are to initiate antihypertensive treatment of systolic blood pressures greater than or equal to 150 mm Hg or greater than or equal to 100 mm Hg diastolic.[31]

Although angiotension receptor blockers are commonly used in nongravid patients with hypertension, this class of medications is contraindicated during pregnancy due to their effects on renal development and intrauterine growth retardation. Based on a recent retrospective cohort study examining the use of antihypertensives in gravid patients with hypertension, superiority of any one particular class of antihypertensives could be made. Both methyldopa and atenolol increase the incidence of fetal low birth weight and intrauterine growth restriction.[32] Current recommendations are to initiate antihypertensive therapy with labetalol, nifedipine, or methyldopa.[2]

Anesthesia Implications

Neuraxial anesthesia

Current guidelines support placing spinal or epidural catheter early for preeclamptic patients to reduce the need for general anesthesia in an emergency requiring urgent delivery.[33] Unless contraindicated, the preferred method of analgesia for both laboring patients and cesarean section is neuraxial anesthesia.[34] The incidence of major complications with placement of neuraxial anesthesia in pregnant women is approximately 1/25,000 for epidural and 1/20,000 to 1/300,000 for spinal anesthesia.[35] There are no large randomized, multicenter studies that indicate increase incidence of complication in preeclamptic patients.

In the setting of preeclampsia, coagulopathy is usually due to thrombocytopenia and, less likely, disseminated intravascular coagulation. The incidence of thrombocytopenia with platelet counts of less than $100 \times 10^9/L$ is approximately 11.6% in patients with pregnancy-induced hypertension.[36] Safe platelet count thresholds to place spinal anesthesia or lumbar epidural catheters have not been set by guidelines.[33] Current standard of practice is using the lower limit of platelet count of 100,000/μL in healthy and preeclamptic pregnant women. In the absence of other coagulation disturbances in preeclamptic patients, case reports reveal less likelihood of neuraxial anesthesia complications with platelet counts of greater than 75,000/μL to 80,000/μL.[37] There are multiple case reports of epidural placements with platelet counts below 75,000/μL, even as low as 20,000/μL, without evidence of spinal hematoma. A multisite retrospective cohort study published in 2015 examined the risk of spinal hematoma after neuraxial placement in thrombocytopenic parturients. The study examined 102 cases and did not find one incidence of spinal hematoma. When the study included case series (n = 499), the risk of spinal hematoma was 0% to 0.6% compared with series morbidity rates of 6.5% for the thrombocytopenic patients who received general anesthesia.[38]

Hypotension induced by spinal anesthesia is caused by sympathetic blockade leading to decrease in uteroplacental blood flow, which may lead to fetal distress. The incidence of spinal-induced hypotension has been found less in preeclamptic patients compared with healthy term parturients.[39,40] One randomized, multicenter study published in 2005 comparing spinal and epidural anesthesia in severe preeclamptic patients found higher incidence of hypotension in the spinal group (51% vs 23%).[34] Hypotension, however, in all groups was easily treated, was of short duration, and did not lead to changes in maternal or neonatal outcomes. Another case cohort published in 2005 compared spinal-induced hypotension between patients with severe preeclampsia and healthy preterm women undergoing cesarean section.[41] Hypotension was defined as a need for ephedrine when there was a 30% decrease in mean arterial pressure or systolic blood pressure below 100 mm Hg. The incidence of hypotension was less in the preeclampsia group (24.6% vs 40.8%). The smaller size of the preeclamptic uterus leading to reduced aortocaval compression was thought to play a role in decreased incidence of hypotension but the current theory is pointing toward preeclampsia-associated factors.[39,41]

General anesthesia

General anesthesia and neuraxial anesthesia have similar complications rates in patients with severe preeclampsia.[42] General anesthesia is used when the preeclamptic patients present with eclampsia, pulmonary edema, depressed levels of consciousness, or signs or symptoms of cerebral edema. Given the risk of direct maternal complications and mortality, such as stroke and cardiac failure, close attention is needed in preventing the exacerbation of hypertension in response to intubation. Esmolol, nitroglycerin, fentanyl, remifentanil, and propofol are all reasonable choices to ablate the response. Magnesium bolus, lidocaine, calcium channel antagonists other than nicardipine, and hydralazine are not recommended.[43,44] Further vigilance is needed and steps should be taken to avoid complications on emergence, such as hypertension, aspiration, and acute pulmonary edema.

Role of invasive monitoring

Current guidelines do not recommend the routine use of invasive hemodynamic monitoring for preeclamptic patients. The decision to use invasive monitoring should be based on their medical comorbidities and cardiovascular risk factors.[29] Patients with mild preeclampsia should have their blood pressure monitored every hour during labor, whereas patients with severe eclampsia should have continuous monitoring. Invasive intra-arterial monitoring may also aid in obtaining frequent blood samples to assess the status of electrolytes, respiratory function, acid-bases balance, and hemotological and liver abnormalities.[45] The incidence of complications, including infection and thrombosis, from arterial catherization is known to be low with proper placement and use.[46] There are no data on the specific risks to paturient patients.

Central venous catheters and pulmonary artery catheters (PACs) are rarely placed for hemodynamic monitoring of preeclamptic patients. Placements of these catheters allow for central venous pressure monitoring, venous access, medication administration, and hemodynamic monitoring. The complication rate associated with central venous catheter placement during pregnancy and postpartum was found to have an overall incidence of 25%, with 12% having an infectious etiology.[47] Complications also included mechanical failure, line infections, superficial and deep thrombosis, hematoma, ventricular tachycardia, and patient discomfort. There is a lack of randomized controlled trials supporting the utility of placing PACs. The complication rate associated with PACs in severe preeclamptic and eclamptic patients is 4%, including venous thrombosis and cellulitis.[48]

ECLAMPSIA – PREVENTION AND MANAGEMENT

Eclampsia is the severe manifestation of the underlying physiologic processes seen in preeclampsia and contributes to maternal morbidity and mortality. Women who have experienced preeclampsia demonstrate white matter lesions on cerebral MRI scans at higher incidence than nonpreeclamptic patients. Moreover, women who have experienced eclampsia have similar lesions for years after the event.[49] Magnesium sulfate is the most effective agent to prevent seizures in women with eclampsia.[50–52]

The mechanism by which magnesium sulfate prevents eclampsia is unclear. The first proposed mechanism is that magnesium acts as a calcium antagonist, decreasing intracellular calcium, and subsequently causing arterial vasodilation and reducing vasospasm.[53] This explanation is not complete, however, because there is MRI evidence that cerebral blood flow is unchanged after a loading dose of magnesium sulfate in preeclamptic women.[54] A competing theory of magnesium's effects are based on the fact that magnesium sulfate decreases blood-brain barrier permeability and subsequently decreases cerebral edema.[55] The final proposed mechanism for the action of magnesium sulfate is through antagonism of the N-methyl-D-aspartate receptor.[56]

Because excessive serum concentrations of magnesium sulfate can lead to respiratory and cardiac depression and death, careful loading and close monitoring are essential. There is no one magnesium dosing regimen that is widely accepted as standard of care. Commonly described regimens include a 4 g to 6 g loading dose and 1 g/h to 2 g/h continuous maintenance infusions. These various regimes, however, do not necessarily result in desired serum levels and must be closely monitored.[57]

POSTPARTUM MANAGEMENT

Delivery of the fetus allows maternal physiology to return toward a mother's baseline. Although there is an initial decline in maternal blood pressure in the first 2 postpartum days, the blood pressure increases again in days 3 to 6. Although a vast majority of cases of preeclampsia present and resolve within 1 week postpartum, it is possible for preeclampsia to present up to 1 month postpartum.

Current recommendations are to monitor preeclamptic women for the first 72 hours and treat hypertension if the systolic blood pressures are greater than or equal to 150 mm Hg or diastolic blood pressures are greater than or equal to 100 mm Hg on 2 or more occasions at least 4 to 6 hours apart. Although furosemide may be more effective than other agents in treating hypertension postpartum, there are few data suggesting improved outcomes.[58–60] Because nonsteroidal anti-inflammatories can worsen hypertension, current recommendations are to avoid them in patients who have been hypertensive for more than 1 day postpartum. Finally, magnesium sulfate therapy should be initiated for at least 24 hours in postpartum patients who present with preeclampsia or hypertension and persistent visual changes or headache.[61]

LONG-TERM OUTCOMES

Approximately 39% of patients diagnosed with preeclampsia have hypertension and approximately 20% have proteinuria 3 months postpartum; 10% to 15% of patients continue to have proteinuria 1 year postpartum.[62] Development of preeclampsia is a major risk factor for postpartum cardiomyopathy.[63,64] Additionally, women who develop preeclampsia are at increased risk for end-stage renal disease.[65,66] Women who develop preeclampsia and become normotensive in subsequent pregnancies are at higher risk of death more than 20 years postpartum.[63] This is presumably due to systemic oxidative injuries sustained during her pregnancy.

In 1 retrospective cohort study comparing 10-year outcomes in women who had preeclampsia versus women who did not, women with preeclampsia had a 15.8-times greater incidence of chronic hypertension. Additionally, women who had preeclampsia had a 1.3-times greater rate of hospitalizations versus those women who did not have preeclampsia.[67] Other cohort studies have similarly seen an increase in the incidence of hypertension as well as an increase in later development of type 2 diabetes mellitus.[68]

FUTURE DEVELOPMENTS

Current research is focused on replacing the angiogenic factors that are depleted in preeclamptic patients. Among consideration are methods to either replace VEGF or to deplete sFLT-1. Researchers have demonstrated reversal of hypertension and improved renal function in a rat model with induced placental ischemia and hypertension.[69] In a pilot study, 8 women underwent extracorporeal removal of sFLT-1 using dextran sulfate cellulose columns. After demonstration that sFLT-1 decreases in a dose-dependent fashion, 3 additional women presenting with severe preterm preeclampsia underwent additional treatments, resulting in prolongation of pregnancies by an average of 19 days versus the untreated cohort, who remained pregnant for 3.6 days.[70] Future therapeutic research will most likely focus on modulating the balance in angiogenic mediators.

SUMMARY

Gestational hypertension is a significant contributor to maternal and fetal morbidity and mortality. Although the specific series of events leading to the development of preeclampsia is not entirely known, significant insights into the role of the maternal immune system have been identified and may become targets of new therapies for high-risk women in the decades ahead. It is important that clinicians do not underappreciate the significant long-term morbidity to the mother, since preeclampsia is associated with higher lifetime maternal risks for developing hypertension and end-stage renal disease. Although additional outcomes studies examining the role of postpartum antihypertensives are necessary, clinicians should closely monitor at-risk patients and treat with medications they are most familiar with.

REFERENCES

1. Brown MA, Lindheimer MD, de Swiet M, et al. The classification and diagnosis of the hypertensive disorders of pregnancy: statement from the international society for the study of hypertension in pregnancy (ISSHP). Hypertens Pregnancy 2001; 20(1):ix–xiv.
2. American College of Obstetricians and Gynecologists, Task Force on Hypertension in Pregnancy. Hypertension in pregnancy. Report of the American College of Obstetricians and Gynecologists' task force on hypertension in pregnancy. Obstet Gynecol 2013;122(5):1122.
3. Lisonkova S, Joseph K. Incidence of preeclampsia: risk factors and outcomes associated with early-versus late-onset disease. Am J Obstet Gynecol 2013; 209(6):544.e1-12.
4. Ros HS, Cnattingius S, Lipworth L. Comparison of risk factors for preeclampsia and gestational hypertension in a population-based cohort study. Am J Epidemiol 1998;147(11):1062–70.
5. World Health Organization. World health report: make every mother and child count. Geneva (Switzerland): World Health Organization; 2005.
6. MacKay AP, Berg CJ, Atrash HK. Pregnancy-related mortality from preeclampsia and eclampsia. Obstet Gynecol 2001;97(4):533–8.
7. Duckitt K, Harrington D. Risk factors for pre-eclampsia at antenatal booking: systematic review of controlled studies. BMJ 2005;330(7491):565.
8. Skupski DW, Nelson S, Kowalik A, et al. Multiple gestations from in vitro fertilization: successful implantation alone is not associated with subsequent preeclampsia. Am J Obstet Gynecol 1996;175(4):1029–32.
9. Garner PR, D'Alton ME, Dudley DK, et al. Preeclampsia in diabetic pregnancies. Am J Obstet Gynecol 1990;163(2):505–8.
10. Sibai BM, Mercer B, Sarinoglu C. Severe preeclampsia in the second trimester: recurrence risk and long-term prognosis. Am J Obstet Gynecol 1991;165(4): 1408–12.
11. Ødegård RA, Vatten LJ, Nilsen ST, et al. Risk factors and clinical manifestations of pre-eclampsia. BJOG 2000;107(11):1410–6.
12. Poon L, Kametas N, Chelemen T, et al. Maternal risk factors for hypertensive disorders in pregnancy: a multivariate approach. J Hum Hypertens 2010;24(2):104–10.
13. Whitley GSJ, Cartwright JE. Trophoblast-mediated spiral artery remodelling: a role for apoptosis. J Anat 2009;215(1):21–6.
14. Tessier DR, Yockell-Lelièvre J, Gruslin A. Uterine spiral artery remodeling: the role of uterine natural killer cells and extravillous trophoblasts in normal and high-risk human pregnancies. Am J Reprod Immunol 2015;74(1):1–11.

15. Burton G, Woods A, Jauniaux E, et al. Rheological and physiological consequences of conversion of the maternal spiral arteries for uteroplacental blood flow during human pregnancy. Placenta 2009;30(6):473–82.

16. Ramsey EM, Crosby RW, Donner MW. Placental vasculature and circulation anatomy, physiology, radiology, clinical aspects: atlas and textbook. Philadelphia: Saunders; 1980.

17. Adamsons K, Myers R. Circulation in the intervillous space: obstetrical considerations in fetal deprivation. In: Gruenwald P, editor. The placental and its maternal supply line. Lancaster: Medical and Technical Publishing; 1975. p. 158–77.

18. Hung T-H, Skepper JN, Burton GJ. In vitro ischemia-reperfusion injury in term human placenta as a model for oxidative stress in pathological pregnancies. Am J Pathol 2001;159(3):1031–43.

19. Rodgers GM, Taylor RN, Roberts JM. Preeclampsia is associated with a serum factor cytotoxic to human endothelial cells. Am J Obstet Gynecol 1988;159(4):908–14.

20. Myers J, Mires G, Macleod M, et al. In preeclampsia, the circulating factors capable of altering in vitro endothelial function precede clinical disease. Hypertension 2005;45(2):258–63.

21. Maynard SE, Min J-Y, Merchan J, et al. Excess placental soluble fms-like tyrosine kinase 1 (sFlt1) may contribute to endothelial dysfunction, hypertension, and proteinuria in preeclampsia. J Clin Invest 2003;111(5):649–58.

22. Ahmad S, Ahmed A. Elevated placental soluble vascular endothelial growth factor receptor-1 inhibits angiogenesis in preeclampsia. Circ Res 2004;95(9):884–91.

23. Levine RJ, Lam C, Qian C, et al. Soluble endoglin and other circulating antiangiogenic factors in preeclampsia. N Engl J Med 2006;355(10):992–1005.

24. Duley L, Henderson-Smart DJ, Meher S, et al. Antiplatelet agents for preventing pre-eclampsia and its complications. Cochrane Database Syst Rev 2007;(2):CD004659.

25. Roberts JM, Myatt L, Spong CY, et al. Vitamins C and E to prevent complications of pregnancy-associated hypertension. N Engl J Med 2010;362(14):1282–91.

26. Rumbold A, Duley L, Crowther C, et al. Antioxidants for preventing pre-eclampsia. Cochrane Database Syst Rev 2008;(1):CD004227.

27. Wagner CL, McNeil R, Hamilton SA, et al. A randomized trial of vitamin D supplementation in 2 community health center networks in South Carolina. Am J Obstet Gynecol 2013;208(2):137.e1-13.

28. Makrides M, Crosby DD, Bain E, et al. Magnesium supplementation in pregnancy. The Cochrane Library; 2014.

29. De-Regil LM, Palacios C, Ansary A, et al. Vitamin D supplementation for women during pregnancy. Cochrane Database Syst Rev 2012;(2):CD008873.

30. Abalos E, Duley L, Steyn D. Antihypertensive drug therapy for mild to moderate hypertension during pregnancy [review]. Cochrane Database Syst Rev 2014;(2):CD002252.

31. National Institute for Clinical Excellence. Hypertension in pregnancy: The management of hypertensive disorders during pregnancy (clinical guideline 107). 2010.

32. Orbach H, Matok I, Gorodischer R, et al. Hypertension and antihypertensive drugs in pregnancy and perinatal outcomes. Am J Obstet Gynecol 2013;208(4):301.e1-6.

33. American Society of Anesthesiologists Task Force on Obstetric Anesthesia. Practice guidelines for obstetric anesthesia: an updated report by the American

society of anesthesiologists task force on obstetric anesthesia. Anesthesiology 2007;106(4):843.

34. Visalyaputra S, Rodanant O, Somboonviboon W, et al. Spinal versus epidural anesthesia for cesarean delivery in severe preeclampsia: a prospective randomized, multicenter study. Anesth Analg 2005;101(3):862–8.

35. Moen V, Dahlgren N, Irestedt L. Severe neurological complications after central neuraxial blockades in Sweden 1990–1999. Anesthesiology 2004;101(4):950–9.

36. Romero R, Mazor M, Lockwood CJ, et al. Clinical significance, prevalence, and natural history of thrombocytopenia in pregnancy-induced hypertension. Am J Perinatol 1989;6(1):32–8.

37. Van Veen JJ, Nokes TJ, Makris M. The risk of spinal haematoma following neuraxial anaesthesia or lumbar puncture in thrombocytopenic individuals. Br J Haematol 2010;148(1):15–25.

38. Goodier CG, Lu JT, Hebbar L, et al. Neuraxial anesthesia in parturients with thrombocytopenia: a multisite retrospective cohort study. Anesth Analg 2015; 121(4):988–91.

39. Aya AG, Mangin R, Vialles N, et al. Patients with severe preeclampsia experience less hypotension during spinal anesthesia for elective cesarean delivery than healthy parturients: a prospective cohort comparison. Anesth Analg 2003; 97(3):867–72.

40. Henke VG, Bateman BT, Leffert LR. Spinal anesthesia in severe preeclampsia. Anesth Analg 2013;117(3):686–93.

41. Aya AG, Vialles N, Tanoubi I, et al. Spinal anesthesia-induced hypotension: a risk comparison between patients with severe preeclampsia and healthy women undergoing preterm cesarean delivery. Anesth Analg 2005;101(3):869–75.

42. Wallace DH, Leveno KJ, Cunningham FG, et al. Randomized comparison of general and regional anesthesia for cesarean delivery in pregnancies complicated by severe preeclampsia. Obstet Gynecol 1995;86(2):193–9.

43. Pant M, Fong R, Scavone B. Prevention of peri-induction hypertension in preeclamptic patients: a focused review. Anesth Analg 2014;119(6):1350–6.

44. Yoo K, Kang D, Jeong H, et al. A dose–response study of remifentanil for attenuation of the hypertensive response to laryngoscopy and tracheal intubation in severely preeclamptic women undergoing caesarean delivery under general anaesthesia. Int J Obstet Anesth 2013;22(1):10–8.

45. Frezza EE, Mezghebe H. Indications and complications of arterial catheter use in surgical or medical intensive care units: analysis of 4932 patients. Am Surg 1998; 64(2):127.

46. Lorente L, Santacreu R, Martín MM, et al. Arterial catheter-related infection of 2,949 catheters. Crit Care 2006;10(3):R83.

47. Nuthalapaty FS, Beck MM, Mabie WC. Complications of central venous catheters during pregnancy and postpartum: a case series. Am J Obstet Gynecol 2009; 201(3):311.e1-5.

48. Gilbert WM, Towner DR, Field NT, et al. The safety and utility of pulmonary artery catheterization in severe preeclampsia and eclampsia. Am J Obstet Gynecol 2000;182(6):1397–403.

49. Aukes A, De Groot JC, Wiegman M, et al. Long-term cerebral imaging after preeclampsia. BJOG 2012;119(9):1117–22.

50. Duley L, Henderson-Smart DJ, Chou D. Magnesium sulphate versus phenytoin for eclampsia. Cochrane Database Syst Rev 2010;(10):CD000128.

51. Duley L, Henderson-Smart DJ, Walker G, et al. Magnesium sulphate versus diazepam for eclampsia. Cochrane Database Syst Rev 2010;(12):CD000127.

52. Belfort MA, Anthony J, Saade GR, et al. A comparison of magnesium sulfate and nimodipine for the prevention of eclampsia. N Engl J Med 2003;348(4):304–11.
53. Euser AG, Cipolla MJ. Resistance artery vasodilation to magnesium sulfate during pregnancy and the postpartum state. Am J Physiol Heart Circ Physiol 2005;288(4):H1521–5.
54. Hatab MR, Zeeman GG, Twickler DM. The effect of magnesium sulfate on large cerebral artery blood flow in preeclampsia. J Matern Fetal Neonatal Med 2005; 17(3):187–92.
55. Euser AG, Bullinger L, Cipolla MJ. Magnesium sulphate treatment decreases blood–brain barrier permeability during acute hypertension in pregnant rats. Exp Physiol 2008;93(2):254–61.
56. Shimosawa I, Takano K, Ando K, et al. Magnesium inhibits norepinephrine release by blocking N-type calcium channels at peripheral sympathetic nerve endings. Hypertension 2004;44(6):897–902.
57. Okusanya B, Oladapo O, Long Q, et al. Clinical pharmacokinetic properties of magnesium sulphate in women with pre-eclampsia and eclampsia: a systematic review. BJOG 2016;123(3):356–66.
58. Tan LK, De Swiet M. The management of postpartum hypertension. BJOG 2002; 109(7):733–6.
59. Magee L, von Dadelszen P. Prevention and treatment of postpartum hypertension. Cochrane Database Syst Rev 2013;(4):CD004351.
60. Podymow T, August P. Postpartum course of gestational hypertension and preeclampsia. Hypertens Pregnancy 2010;29(3):294–300.
61. Sibai BM. Etiology and management of postpartum hypertension-preeclampsia. Am J Obstet Gynecol 2012;206(6):470–5.
62. Berks D, Steegers EA, Molas M, et al. Resolution of hypertension and proteinuria after preeclampsia. Obstet Gynecol 2009;114(6):1307–14.
63. Funai EF, Friedlander Y, Paltiel O, et al. Long-term mortality after preeclampsia. Epidemiology 2005;16(2):206–15.
64. Patten IS, Rana S, Shahul S, et al. Cardiac angiogenic imbalance leads to peripartum cardiomyopathy. Nature 2012;485(7398):333–8.
65. Vikse BE, Irgens LM, Leivestad T, et al. Preeclampsia and the risk of end-stage renal disease. N Engl J Med 2008;359(8):800–9.
66. Wang I-K, Muo C-H, Chang Y-C, et al. Association between hypertensive disorders during pregnancy and end-stage renal disease: a population-based study. Can Med Assoc J 2013;185(3):207–13.
67. Shalom G, Shoham-Vardi I, Sergienko R, et al. Is preeclampsia a significant risk factor for long-term hospitalizations and morbidity? J Matern Fetal Neonatal Med 2013;26(1):13–5.
68. Lykke JA, Langhoff-Roos J, Sibai BM, et al. Hypertensive pregnancy disorders and subsequent cardiovascular morbidity and type 2 diabetes mellitus in the mother. Hypertension 2009;53(6):944–51.
69. Gilbert JS, Verzwyvelt J, Colson D, et al. Recombinant vascular endothelial growth factor 121 infusion lowers blood pressure and improves renal function in rats with placentalischemia-induced hypertension. Hypertension 2010;55(2): 380–5.
70. Thadhani R, Kisner T, Hagmann H, et al. Pilot study of extracorporeal removal of soluble fms-like tyrosine kinase 1 in preeclampsia. Circulation 2011;124(8): 940–50.

Optimal Pain Management After Cesarean Delivery

 CrossMark

Caitlin Dooley Sutton, MD, Brendan Carvalho, MBBCh, FRCA*

KEYWORDS

- Cesarean delivery • Pain management • Intrathecal opioids • Multimodal analgesia

KEY POINTS

- Effective pain management is a key priority of women undergoing cesarean delivery, and severe postoperative pain is associated with persistent pain, greater opioid use, delayed functional recovery, and increased postpartum depression.
- Intrathecal morphine is the gold standard for postcesarean pain, providing excellent and prolonged postoperative analgesia.
- Multimodal analgesia should include scheduled nonsteroidal antiinflammatory drugs and acetaminophen, with opioids reserved for severe breakthrough pain.
- Wound infiltration and transversus abdominis plane blocks play an important role in multimodal analgesia for patients who are unable to receive neuraxial opioids or whose pain is not adequately controlled.
- Analgesics can potentially transfer to breastfeeding infants, but transfer can be minimized by careful drug selection and optimal timing of administration.

INTRODUCTION

The rate of cesarean delivery in the United States has been increasing over the past decades and now exceeds 32% of births.[1] Effective postoperative analgesia is critical, because women who undergo cesarean delivery rank avoidance of pain during and after surgery as their highest priority.[2] Management of postcesarean pain may have lasting effects, and severe acute postoperative pain is associated with persistent pain, greater opioid use, delayed functional recovery, and increased postpartum depression.[3] Effective pain relief after cesarean delivery improves a woman's ability to function and interact with her newborn infant.[4]

An individual patient's specific plan should be determined in the context of any medical and psychiatric comorbidities, chronic pain, and prior postoperative or postpartum experiences.[5] The American Pain Society recommends that planning for

Disclosure Statement: The authors have nothing to disclose.
Department of Anesthesiology, Perioperative and Pain Medicine, Stanford University School of Medicine, 300 Pasteur Drive, Stanford, CA 94305, USA
* Corresponding author.
E-mail address: bcarvalho@stanford.edu

Anesthesiology Clin 35 (2017) 107–124
http://dx.doi.org/10.1016/j.anclin.2016.09.010   anesthesiology.theclinics.com

postoperative pain management should begin in the preoperative period. Physicians should focus on individualizing perioperative pain management, often through a multi-modal approach.[5] Compared with other surgeries, formulating a plan for optimal anesthesia and analgesia for cesarean delivery involves several distinct considerations:

- Surgical anesthesia is almost exclusively neuraxial and is performed in awake, unsedated patients
- Preemptive analgesic use is limited because of concerns for in-utero fetal drug transfer
- The potential transfer of analgesic drugs to breastfeeding neonates should be considered
- Maximal postoperative mobility of mothers in order to facilitate optimal neonatal care is extremely important

Multimodal analgesia options for providing optimal postoperative pain relief for women undergoing uncomplicated cesarean delivery with neuraxial anesthesia are summarized in this article. Analgesic options are appropriate for most parturients, but there are many women whose medical comorbidities require special consideration. Conditions that require alterations to pain management include chronic pain, obstructive sleep apnea, and a contraindication to neuraxial anesthesia. Although several key points are highlighted, detailed management of these conditions is beyond the scope of this article.

NEURAXIAL MEDICATIONS

- Intrathecal morphine
- Epidural morphine
- Intrathecal hydromorphone
- Continuous and patient-controlled epidural infusions
- Nonopioid neuraxial adjuncts

The American Society of Anesthesiology's Obstetric Anesthesia Practice Guidelines and the American Pain Society's Clinical Practice Guidelines both recommend the routine use of neuraxial anesthesia for cesarean delivery.[5,6] The use of neuraxial anesthesia for cesarean delivery is promoted because of decreased maternal risk and improved fetal outcomes, but the additional benefit of superior postoperative analgesia with the use of neuraxial opioids deserves emphasis.[7]

Standard regimens for intraoperative cesarean anesthesia consist of a combination of local anesthetic and a lipophilic opioid (eg, fentanyl). Although neither drug provides prolonged postoperative analgesia,[8] they provide analgesia in the early postoperative recovery period until the onset of longer-acting neuraxial opioids; neuraxial morphine has an analgesic onset of approximately 60 to 90 minutes.

Intrathecal Morphine

Intrathecal morphine is the gold standard single-shot drug for postcesarean pain, providing long-lasting analgesia for 14 to 36 hours.[8,9] The optimal dose of intrathecal morphine appropriate for all patients has not been determined. Variations in dose seem to be more closely related to duration of analgesia as opposed to more effective pain relief or less opioid use. A recent meta-analysis showed that higher doses (>100 µg) of intrathecal morphine prolong analgesia by a mean difference of 4.5 hours, with time to first request for additional analgesia of 9.7 to 26.6 hours for doses of 50 to 100 µg versus 13.8 to 39.5 hours for doses greater than 100 to 250 µg.[9] Pain scores and opioid use in the first 24 hours after cesarean delivery were similar between groups. However, higher doses present a trade-off of longer analgesic duration versus increased side effects of nausea, vomiting, and pruritus. Side effects can be minimized with the selection of an appropriate dose of intrathecal morphine, as well as with appropriate prophylactic and treatment strategies (**Table 1**). Patients experience

Table 1
Prevention and treatment of neuraxial morphine side effects

Side Effect	Prophylaxis Strategies	Treatment Options
Nausea and vomiting	Use low doses (eg, ≤150 μg intrathecal morphine) Unimodal options[93–95]: • Ondansetron 4–8 mg IV • Metoclopramide 10 mg IV • Dexamethasone 4–8 mg IV • Droperidol 0.625 mg IV • Scopolamine 1.5 mg patch Combination of drugs for improved efficacy[97]: • Ondansetron 4 mg IV + metoclopramide 10 mg IV • Dexamethasone 8 mg IV + droperidol 0.625 mg IV	Ideally use a drug with a different mechanism of action than was used for prophylaxis[92] Treatment options[96]: • Ondansetron 4–8 mg IV • Metoclopramide 10 mg IV • Propofol 10–20 mg IV • Promethazine 6.25–12.5 mg IV
Pruritus	Use low doses (eg, ≤150 μg intrathecal morphine) Ondansetron 4–8 mg IV may reduce incidence, severity, and need for rescue treatment[102] Pretreatment with nalbuphine or naloxone is not effective[103]	Treatment options[98–101]: • Nalbuphine 2.5–5 mg IV • Naloxone 100–200 μg IV • Ondansetron 4–8 mg IV • Butorphanol 1 mg IV, infusion of 0.2 mg/h • Pentazocine 15 mg IV Treatment comparisons[101,104]: • Nalbuphine has better efficacy than naloxone • Pentazocine is more effective than ondansetron
Respiratory depression	Use low doses; eg, ≤150 μg intrathecal morphine Identify patients at risk[106,107]: • Obstructive sleep apnea • Obesity • Chronic pain/opioid tolerance Caution if receiving sedating drugs • Magnesium sulfate • Diphenhydramine • Promethazine	Naloxone bolus followed by low-dose naloxone infusion to avoid recurrence of respiratory depression and minimize pain from opioid antagonism[105] Supplemental oxygen only for treatment because prophylactic oxygen may mask respiratory depression

Abbreviation: IV, intravenous.

a lower incidence of nausea/vomiting (odds ratio [OR], 0.44 [0.27, 0.73]) and pruritus (OR, 0.34 [0.20, 0.59]) when receiving lower (50–100 μg) versus higher (>100–250 μg) intrathecal morphine doses.[9] Importantly, none of the studies in this meta-analysis reported respiratory depression in any patient. Although women with obstructive sleep apnea and morbid obesity are potentially at increased risk for respiratory depression,[10] intrathecal and epidural morphine should not be avoided in these patients, because neuraxial opioids provide greater analgesic efficacy at a lesser risk of respiratory depression than intravenous opioids.

Epidural Morphine

Although most elective cesarean deliveries in the United States are performed with spinal anesthesia,[11] unplanned cesarean deliveries are often performed on laboring patients with epidurals in situ. For these patients, epidural catheters can be used for administration of epidural morphine for postoperative analgesia. The optimal dose is 2 to 4 mg, with larger doses not definitively providing superior analgesia.[7,12] Studies that have compared epidural with intrathecal morphine have found similar analgesic efficacy and side effects.[13,14] However, intrathecal morphine is generally preferred to epidural administration given its lower opioid dose and therefore less potential neonatal drug transfer.

Intrathecal Hydromorphone

With recent shortages of preservative-free morphine in the United States, providers have gained more experience with the use of intrathecal hydromorphone. A recent dose-finding study identified the dose ratio of intrathecal morphine to intrathecal hydromorphone to be 2:1.[15] Both medications provided high patient satisfaction rates, and adverse effects of nausea and pruritus did not differ between groups.[15] Given that morphine is more hydrophilic, morphine is anticipated to have a longer duration of analgesia after single-dose administration compared with hydromorphone.

Continuous and Patient-Controlled Epidural Infusions

Although continuous and patient-controlled epidural analgesia infusions have been used for postcesarean analgesia, their use decreases maternal mobility, complicates anticoagulation prophylaxis, increases nursing workload, and adds to cost.[16] For most young, healthy women desiring a timely recovery to baseline activity after uncomplicated cesarean delivery, the marginal benefits compared with single-shot intrathecal or epidural opioids given at the time of surgery do not warrant the routine use of continuous epidural infusion after cesarean delivery. However, these epidural catheter-based techniques should be considered in special circumstances (eg, women with chronic pain).

Nonopioid Neuraxial Adjuncts

Neuraxial clonidine may improve postcesarean analgesia when used as an adjunct to local anesthetics and opioids, but it is associated with hypotension and sedation.[17] A black box warning noting the risk of hemodynamic instability in obstetric, postpartum, and perioperative patients highlights the need for special consideration before use of this drug.[18] If used, clonidine should be reserved for patients at high risk for uncontrolled postoperative pain, such as those with a history of poorly controlled postoperative pain or chronic pain. Neostigmine has historically not been recommended for neuraxial administration because of the high incidence of nausea.[17] The 2016 American Pain Society guidelines for postoperative pain management recommend against the use of neostigmine as a neuraxial adjuvant medication, citing a lack of clear benefit and insufficient evidence of safety.[5]

ORAL AND INTRAVENOUS ANALGESIC ADJUVANTS

- Acetaminophen
- Nonsteroidal antiinflammatory drugs (NSAIDs)
- Combining acetaminophen and NSAIDs
- Dexamethasone
- Gabapentinoids
- Ketamine
- Opioids

Neuraxial opioids provide the greatest analgesic effect size for post–cesarean delivery pain management, but most women still require additional analgesia. Supplemental nonopioid medications should be used to improve analgesia and decrease the side effects of opioids. Minimizing the use of intravenous and oral opioids with nonopioid medication is particularly critical, because up to 1 in 300 opioid-naive women become persistent users of opioids after cesarean delivery.[19] Through distinct mechanisms at multiple receptor sites, multimodal analgesia has been associated with superior pain relief and decreased opioid use compared with the use of a single analgesic.[20,21]

Acetaminophen

Acetaminophen is used extensively in the postoperative period and provides an opioid-sparing effect of approximately 20%.[22] Its ability to provide effective analgesia with minimal adverse effects[23] supports the routine use of scheduled acetaminophen for 2 to 3 days after cesarean delivery. In 2009, the US Food and Drug Administration changed the recommended maximum daily dose of acetaminophen from 4000 mg to 3250 mg.[24] Avoiding opioid/acetaminophen combination pills is recommended in order to decrease unnecessary opioid use and avoid exceeding recommended maximum doses of acetaminophen.[25]

Nonsteroidal Antiinflammatory Drugs

NSAIDs are a key component of multimodal postoperative pain management. NSAIDs decrease pain scores, particularly related to visceral cramping pain. They have a 30% to 50% opioid-sparing effect,[20,26] and therefore can reduce the incidence of opioid-related side effects.[21,27] The use of nonselective NSAIDs has been associated with a statistically significant increase in surgical bleeding,[26] and they should be used cautiously in patients at increased risk for bleeding. Evidence does not show an effect of NSAIDs on cardiovascular events, gastrointestinal bleeding, or renal impairment in patients with normal preoperative renal function, but clinicians should consider these potential NSAID effects in at-risk patients (eg, women with preeclampsia with renal impairment).[23] For healthy patients with good intraoperative hemostasis, NSAIDs should be given routinely in the immediate postpartum period. No studies have evaluated the relative efficacy of one NSAID compared with another, so use can be based on drug availability and breastfeeding safety data.

Selective cyclooxygenase (COX) 2 inhibitors such as celecoxib were designed to decrease the gastrointestinal and hematologic risks associated with nonselective NSAIDs. To date, no trials have compared the outcomes of selective versus nonselective NSAIDs for cesarean delivery analgesia. Studies of COX2 inhibitors for post–cesarean delivery analgesia have shown limited analgesic efficacy,[28] and their use should be reserved for patients who are intolerant of nonselective NSAIDs.[5]

Combining Acetaminophen and Nonsteroidal Antiinflammatory Drugs

Acetaminophen and NSAIDs are more effective when used together and should be used in combination for postcesarean analgesia in patients without contraindications.[29] Staggered dosing of around-the-clock acetaminophen and NSAIDs increases the number of patient interruptions and increases nursing workload without proven benefit, so consideration should be given to administering the two drugs simultaneously at set time points (eg, every 6 hours). Given the higher cost and lack of clear evidence for improved analgesia, intravenous administration of NSAIDs and acetaminophen is not recommended compared with oral administration.[30] However, intravenous formulations offer a good alternative for patients not yet tolerating oral intake or experiencing nausea or vomiting.

Dexamethasone

Glucocorticoids have analgesic and antiemetic properties in addition to their antiinflammatory effects. The use of a single perioperative dose of dexamethasone has been shown to improve pain relief compared with placebo for patients undergoing surgery under general anesthesia, but is associated with marginally higher blood glucose levels at 24 hours postoperatively and should be avoided in patients with insulin resistance.[31] Wound healing and infection rates have not been found to be increased after single-dose perioperative dexamethasone administration.[31,32] For patients undergoing cesarean delivery under spinal anesthesia using low-dose intrathecal morphine, a single dose of dexamethasone before surgery significantly decreased the incidence of nausea and vomiting and improved analgesia on the first postoperative day.[33] Doses between 1.25 and 20 mg have been described, and the optimal dose has not been determined.[31]

Gabapentinoids

Although more commonly used in the management of chronic pain, gabapentin has an analgesic and opioid-sparing effect in the acute postoperative period.[34] Gabapentin has also been shown to decrease opioid-associated vomiting and pruritus,[34] but the drug has its own side effects, especially sedation (Number needed to harm [NNH] = 8–35) and dizziness (NNH = 12).[34,35] Initial enthusiasm for a single preoperative dose of gabapentin 600 mg to decrease postcesarean pain and increase maternal satisfaction[36] has been tempered by subsequent studies that did not show a significant analgesic effect.[37] Even a 2-day perioperative course of gabapentin did not improve postcesarean analgesia and was associated with increased sedation.[38] The use of pregabalin for postcesarean analgesia has not been studied, and doses of 75 and 150 mg did not reduce opioid use after abdominal hysterectomy.[39] Pregabalin administration in the perioperative period has been associated with side effects such as visual disturbances and dizziness.[40,41]

Gabapentin is a neurotropic drug and has a high umbilical vein to maternal vein ratio, which limits preemptive administration in the cesarean delivery setting.[36] Breast milk transfer is also a potential concern.[42] Given the lack of strong evidence for significantly improved acute or chronic postoperative pain relief in the cesarean delivery setting, as well as the potential adverse effects and unclear neonatal safety profile, gabapentinoids are not recommended for routine postcesarean analgesia. In patients with a history of chronic pain or pain not relieved by standard treatment protocols, gabapentin can be considered as part of a multimodal analgesic regimen to improve pain relief and decrease opioid consumption.

Ketamine

Low-dose ketamine (10–15 mg) has analgesic and opioid-sparing effects in the first 24 hours after nonobstetric surgery and cesarean delivery with general anesthesia.[43] For patients undergoing cesarean delivery with spinal anesthesia using intrathecal morphine, a single dose of ketamine after delivery did not offer any analgesic benefit.[44] However, ketamine has been associated with improved analgesia in patients undergoing cesarean delivery without intrathecal morphine.[45–47] Hallucinations or disturbing dreams associated with low-dose ketamine are reported but are infrequent, whereas complaints of dizziness, lightheadedness, or visual effects are common.[44,45] A single intraoperative dose of ketamine 10 mg has been associated with lower pain scores 2 weeks postpartum,[44] and the drug may have a role in patients at risk for chronic pain after surgery.

Opioids

Opioids should be reserved for treatment of breakthrough pain when pain relief from the combination of neuraxial opioids and nonopioid adjuncts outlined earlier is inadequate. Intravenous opioids have not been found to provide superior analgesia compared with oral opioids, are associated with more side effects, and limit mobility after cesarean delivery[48,49]; therefore, the use of oral opioids is generally preferred. Oxycodone, hydrocodone, and tramadol are oral opioids commonly used in the cesarean delivery setting. Codeine is not recommended because maternal and neonatal pharmacogenomic and metabolic variability can affect both efficacy and side effects.[50] Intravenous opioids should be reserved for patients in extreme pain or intolerant of oral intake. When intravenous opioids are required for a sustained period of time, patient-controlled analgesia (without the use of a basal infusion)[51] is preferable because of greater analgesic efficacy and higher patient satisfaction.[52]

LOCAL ANESTHETICS

- Wound infiltration
- Transversus abdominis plane (TAP) and quadratus lumborum blocks
- Other local anesthetic options

Wound Infiltration

Wound infiltration of local anesthetics is a commonly used method of supplemental analgesia for abdominal surgery.[53] A meta-analysis comparing wound infiltration with epidural analgesia for abdominal surgery showed comparable pain scores at 24 and 48 hours, but the trials included were heterogeneous.[54] Women who undergo cesarean delivery with general anesthesia may benefit from local anesthetics delivered via wound infiltration or TAP block.[55,56] However, in patients who receive spinal anesthesia and neuraxial opioids, the benefit of single-dose local anesthetic wound infiltration is minimal. Single-dose local anesthetic wound infiltration at the time of surgery is unlikely to last beyond the duration of the neuraxial block, affects only somatic (not visceral) pain, and has variable efficacy.[53,57]

Catheter-based local anesthetic instillation has been suggested as an alternative to single-dose infiltration. Continuous wound instillation of local anesthetic reduces pain scores, opioid use, and opioid-related nausea and vomiting for up to 48 hours postoperatively.[53,57,58] However, the analgesia from local anesthetic techniques in isolation is less effective than neuraxial opioids or NSAIDs.[59] If used, wound instillation should be considered part of a multimodal treatment plan, and the catheter should be placed subfascially rather than subcutaneously or suprafascially for optimal efficacy.[60]

Several medications have been studied as possible adjuvants to wound instillation of local anesthetics. Dexamethasone 16 mg added to local anesthetic instilled subcutaneously into the wound prolongs analgesia compared with local anesthetic alone.[61] Diclofenac (300 mg over 48 hours) instilled into cesarean delivery incisions provided more pain relief than the same dose given intravenously.[55] Instillation of magnesium sulfate (750 mg as an adjunct to ropivacaine) prolonged analgesia compared with local anesthetic alone and was not associated with any significant side effects.[62] The addition of ketorolac (30 mg over 48 hours), but not hydromorphone, to local anesthetic wound instillation has been associated with lower levels of inflammatory mediators as well as less pain and analgesic use after cesarean delivery.[63] Studies comparing the safety of wound instillation versus systemic administration of drugs such as NSAIDs or glucocorticoids should be performed before wound instillation of these adjuvant medications can be recommended as standard practice.

Transversus Abdominis Plane and Quadratus Lumborum Blocks

There is no significant analgesic and opioid-sparing benefit of routine TAP block after cesarean delivery in patients who receive intrathecal morphine.[64,65] In patients who undergo general anesthesia or spinal anesthesia without intrathecal or epidural morphine, TAP blocks can significantly improve postoperative pain and reduce opioid consumption.[56,64–66] TAP blocks have been found to provide similar analgesia after cesarean delivery compared with continuous wound site local anesthetic instillation.[67–69] The duration of sensory blockade for single-shot TAP block is limited to 6 to 12 hours, with a mean analgesic effect of 9.5 hours (8.5–11.9 hours).[70] TAP blocks have been used effectively for rescue analgesia in the postanesthesia care unit for patients with severe postoperative incisional pain who are not responding to routine analgesics and rescue opioids.[71] Before using TAP blocks for rescue analgesia, clinicians should evaluate the nature and location of pain because, as with wound infiltration of local anesthetic, TAP blocks are effective primarily for somatic incisional pain rather than visceral or cramping pain. Studies comparing TAP blocks with intrathecal morphine have found that TAP blocks provide inferior analgesia, but they have a lower incidence of opioid-related side effects, such as nausea.[64,65]

Although the addition of sufentanil to TAP block has been shown to decrease opioid requirements after cesarean delivery,[72] fentanyl added to TAP block did not provide additional analgesia compared with systemic administration of the same dose. These conflicting results suggest that systemic absorption may account for the improved analgesia when opioids are added to local anesthetics for TAP block.[73] The addition of clonidine to the local anesthetic in TAP blocks did not improve short-term or long-term cesarean delivery analgesia.[74] On balance, current evidence does not support the use of adjuvants for TAP blocks until safety and efficacy are proved. Larger volumes are associated with greater spread and improve the analgesic effect of TAP blocks.[75] There is concern for local anesthetic toxicity with TAP block,[76] with several cases reported in the setting of cesarean delivery.[67,77] Local anesthetic concentration should be adjusted as necessary to avoid exceeding maximum recommended doses (eg, ropivacaine 0.25% 20–25 mL per side). A recent study evaluating quadratus lumborum block after cesarean delivery with spinal anesthesia (without intrathecal morphine but with a multimodal regimen including acetaminophen and NSAIDs) found reduced opioid requirements and pain scores.[78]

Other Local Anesthetic Options

Liposomal bupivacaine for wound infiltration or TAP blocks has not been evaluated in the cesarean delivery setting. However, subfascial wound infiltration of liposomal bupivacaine after open total abdominal hysterectomy provided superior pain relief at rest and with coughing at 6 hours compared with TAP blocks.[79] The analgesic efficacy and safety of liposomal versus standard bupivacaine for post–cesarean delivery pain must be determined before routine administration can be recommended. Bupivacaine-soaked absorbable gel sponges have been reported to decrease pain scores, analgesic consumption, and side effects after cesarean delivery compared with controls.[80]

NONPHARMACOLOGIC TECHNIQUES

Cognitive and behavioral treatment modalities including guided imagery, hypnosis, and music have limited analgesic effects, but they are noninvasive and lack side effects and therefore can be considered as part of a multimodal analgesic regimen that may reduce anxiety and potentially improve pain.[5,81,82] Transcutaneous electrical nerve stimulation (TENS) is thought to modulate pain by activating descending inhibitory pathways. TENS has been shown to be more effective than placebo stimulation in reducing incisional pain associated with movement, although evidence is insufficient to recommend specific TENS regimens for cesarean pain management.[83] Physicians occasionally recommend the use of abdominal binders after cesarean delivery based on anecdotal reports of improved pain, but a recent randomized controlled trial comparing the use of abdominal binders with controls after cesarean delivery showed no difference in pain scores or postoperative distress.[84]

SUGGESTED ANALGESIC PROTOCOL

Table 2 shows a suggested analgesic protocol for routine cesarean delivery performed with neuraxial anesthesia. Analgesic protocols should include a standard protocol for most patients, with modifications for patients who require general anesthesia, experience severe pain not responding to standard management, or have a preexisting diagnosis of chronic pain. Patient-centered analgesic protocols with various options may provide superior maternal analgesia and satisfaction compared with a one-size-fits-all approach.

BREASTFEEDING CONSIDERATIONS

More than 70% of women in the United States attempt breastfeeding, and the rate continues to increase.[85] Good analgesia promotes successful breastfeeding and maternal-neonatal bonding, but analgesics have the potential to transfer to the breastfeeding infant.[86] Neonatal drug exposure is typically expressed as relative infant dose (RID). The RID takes into account maternal and neonatal weights, and an RID greater than 10% is generally considered a level of concern.[87] **Table 3** shows the RID of analgesics that are commonly used for cesarean delivery pain management.

An in-depth discussion of the physiology and pharmacokinetics of drug transfer through breastfeeding is outlined in several reviews.[86–89] Clinicians should have a basic understanding of breastfeeding physiology when managing post–cesarean delivery analgesia. Postoperative analgesics for women who are breastfeeding should be prescribed with several general principals[86–91] taken into account:

- Opioid-sparing multimodal analgesia is preferable, because opioids are associated with breast milk transfer and may cause neonatal sedation.
- The amount of drug in breast milk parallels maternal blood levels. Clinicians should use the lowest effective dose and administer opioids intrathecally or epidurally rather than intravenously when possible.
- Drugs with a short half-life, inactive metabolites, and long record of safe use are the best choice in this setting.

Table 2
Suggested analgesic protocol for post–cesarean delivery in-hospital pain management

Setting	Drug	Dose and Route	Prescribing Information
Standard care[a] (prescribed at time of surgery)	Neuraxial morphine	Preferred: intrathecal morphine 100–150 μg or epidural morphine 2–3 mg after delivery	With intrathecal hyperbaric bupivacaine 12 mg and fentanyl 15 μg With epidural 2% lidocaine 15–25 mL (±bicarbonate and epinephrine) ± fentanyl 50–100 μg
	NSAIDs	Ibuprofen 600 mg PO (or ketorolac 15 mg IV if NPO)	Every 6 h (scheduled) for 48–72 h after cesarean delivery
	Acetaminophen	Acetaminophen 650 mg PO (or IV if NPO)	Every 6 h (scheduled) for 48–72 h after cesarean delivery
	Oral opioids	Oxycodone 5–10 mg PO	As needed for breakthrough pain: VNPS ≤4/10: 5 mg VNPS >4/10: 10 mg
Ongoing or severe postoperative pain[b]	IV opioids	IV morphine, fentanyl, or hydromorphone	Intermittent IV boluses or IV patient-controlled analgesia
	Regional anesthesia	Bilateral TAP block	0.25% ropivacaine 20–25 mL per side
	Oral adjuvants	Gabapentin	600 mg PO rescue dose (300 mg PO every 8 h for ongoing severe pain)
		Dexamethasone	4–8 mg PO

Based on the analgesic protocol used at Lucile Packard Children's Hospital, Stanford University, California.

Abbreviations: NPO, nil per os, not tolerating oral medication, or vomiting; PO, per os administration; VNPS, verbal numerical pain score (0–10).

[a] For women identified to be at risk for severe postoperative pain (eg, chronic pain, opioid tolerant) consider the following analgesic options: (1) postoperative patient-controlled epidural analgesia with local anesthetic and opioid (preferred) or higher initial dose of intrathecal morphine (200–300 μg). (2) Local anesthetic wound instillation (0.5% ropivacaine 5 mL/h subfascially for 48–72 h after cesarean). (3) Additional adjuvants: subanesthetic ketamine 10 to 15 mg IV and/or dexamethasone 4 to 8 mg IV after delivery of the baby.

[b] Approximately 5% to 10% of patients managed by standard care analgesics listed above may require additional analgesic interventions for breakthrough pain.

- Lipophilic drugs are most likely to cross into the breast milk, whereas highly protein-bound drugs (eg, NSAIDs, local anesthetics) have limited drug transfer.
- Drugs with low oral bioavailability have limited transfer to breastfeeding infants.
- Timing breastfeeding to coincide with maternal blood drug trough levels is optimal if it can be achieved without compromising maternal analgesic needs.
- So-called "pump and dump" is not necessary for routine post–cesarean delivery patients.
- The amount of colostrum in the first few days after delivery is small, so the amount of drug transfer is small compared with several days after birth.
- Women should be informed about potential transfer of pain medications on breastfeeding newborns.

Table 3
Relative infant doses of analgesics commonly used after cesarean delivery

Medication	RID (%)
Acetaminophen[87,88]	1.3–6.4
Ibuprofen[87,88,108]	0.1–0.7
Ketorolac[88,91,108,109]	0.2–0.4
Celecoxib[87,108]	0.3
Dexamethasone	No data
Gabapentin[87,110]	1.3–6.5
Pregabalin	No data
Hydrocodone[86,91]	1.6–3.7
Oxycodone[86,109]	1.5–8
Tramadol[87,111]	2.4–2.9
Fentanyl[88,109]	0.9–3
Morphine[87,88,109]	5.8–10.7

The RID is expressed as a percentage and is weight adjusted for the infant, normalizing that amount of drug to which the neonate is exposed relative to the mother's dose.

SUMMARY

Cesarean delivery rates are increasing worldwide, and effective pain relief is a key priority of women undergoing cesarean delivery. Pain management in women after cesarean delivery is unique among surgeries in that initial anesthesia is almost exclusively neuraxial, preemptive analgesic use is limited by fetal drug transfer, and postoperative analgesics given to the mother have the potential for transfer to the breastfeeding neonate. In addition to pain relief, optimal management of patients after cesarean delivery should address the goals of maximizing maternal mobility and rapid recovery to baseline functionality. Multimodal analgesia should include neuraxial morphine in conjunction with nonopioid adjuncts such as scheduled NSAIDs and acetaminophen, with additional opioids reserved for severe breakthrough pain.

REFERENCES

1. Hamilton BE, Martin JA, Osterman MJK, et al. Births: final data for 2014. Natl Vital Stat Rep 2015;64(12):1–104.
2. Carvalho B, Cohen SE, Lipman SS, et al. Patient preferences for anesthesia outcomes associated with cesarean delivery. Anesth Analg 2005;101(2):1182–7.
3. Eisenach JC, Pan PH, Smiley R, et al. Severity of acute pain after childbirth, but not type of delivery, predicts persistent pain and postpartum depression. Pain 2008;140(1):87–94.
4. Hirose M, Hara Y, Hosokawa T, et al. The effect of postoperative analgesia with continuous epidural bupivacaine after cesarean section on the amount of breast feeding and infant weight gain. Anesth Analg 1996;82(6):1166–9.
5. Chou R, Gordon DB, de Leon-Casasola OA, et al. Management of postoperative pain: a clinical practice guideline from the American Pain Society, the American Society of Regional Anesthesia and Pain Medicine, and the American Society of Anesthesiologists' Committee on Regional Anesthesia, Executive Committee, and Administrative Council. J Pain 2016;17(2):131–57.

6. American Society of Anesthesiologists Task Force on Obstetric Anesthesia. Practice guidelines for obstetric anesthesia: an updated report by the American Society of Anesthesiologists Task Force on Obstetric Anesthesia. Anesthesiology 2007;106(4):843–63.

7. Bonnet M-P, Mignon A, Mazoit J-X, et al. Analgesic efficacy and adverse effects of epidural morphine compared to parenteral opioids after elective caesarean section: a systematic review. Eur J Pain 2010;14(9):894.e1-9.

8. Dahl JB, Jeppesen IS, Jørgensen H, et al. Intraoperative and postoperative analgesic efficacy and adverse effects of intrathecal opioids in patients undergoing cesarean section with spinal anesthesia: a qualitative and quantitative systematic review of randomized controlled trials. Anesthesiology 1999;91(6): 1919–27.

9. Sultan P, Halpern SH, Pushpanathan E, et al. The effect of intrathecal morphine dose on outcomes after elective cesarean delivery: a meta-analysis. Anesth Analg 2016;123(1):154–64.

10. Chan JKW, Leung RCC, Lai CKW. Diagnosis and treatment of obstructive sleep apnea. Clin Pulm Med 1998;5(1):60–8.

11. Traynor AJ, Aragon M, Ghosh D, et al. Obstetric anesthesia workforce survey: a 30-year update. Anesth Analg 2016;122(6):1939–46.

12. Palmer CM, Nogami WM, Alves DM, et al. Postcesarean epidural morphine: a dose-response study. Anesth Analg 2000;90(4):887–91.

13. Dualé C, Frey C, Bolandard F, et al. Epidural versus intrathecal morphine for postoperative analgesia after Caesarean section. Br J Anaesth 2003;91(5): 690–4.

14. Sarvela J, Halonen P, Soikkeli A, et al. A double-blinded, randomized comparison of intrathecal and epidural morphine for elective cesarean delivery. Anesth Analg 2002;95(2):436–40. Table of contents.

15. Sviggum HP, Arendt KW, Jacob AK, et al. Intrathecal hydromorphone and morphine for postcesarean delivery analgesia: determination of the ED90 using a sequential allocation biased-coin method. Anesth Analg 2016;123(3):690–7.

16. Vercauteren M, Vereecken K, La Malfa M, et al. Cost-effectiveness of analgesia after Caesarean section. A comparison of intrathecal morphine and epidural PCA. Acta Anaesthesiol Scand 2002;46(1):85–9.

17. Roelants F. The use of neuraxial adjuvant drugs (neostigmine, clonidine) in obstetrics. Curr Opin Anaesthesiol 2006;19(3):233–7.

18. Clonidine hydrochloride [package insert]. Columbus, OH: PharmaForce; 2009.

19. Bateman BT, Franklin JM, Bykov K, et al. Persistent opioid use following Cesarean delivery: patterns and predictors among opioid naïve women. Am J Obstet Gynecol 2016;215(3):353.e1-18.

20. Elia N, Lysakowski C, Tramer M. Does multimodal analgesia with acetaminophen, nonsteroidal anti-inflammatory drugs, or selective cyclooxygenase-2 inhibitors and patient-controlled analgesia morphine offer advantages over morphine alone? Anesthesiology 2005;103:1296–394.

21. Maund E, McDaid C, Rice S, et al. Paracetamol and selective and non-selective non-steroidal anti-inflammatory drugs for the reduction in morphine-related side-effects after major surgery: a systematic review. Br J Anaesth 2011;106(3): 292–7.

22. Remy C, Marret E, Bonnet F. Effects of acetaminophen on morphine side-effects and consumption after major surgery: meta-analysis of randomized controlled trials. Br J Anaesth 2005;94(4):505–13.

23. Mathiesen O, Wetterslev J, Kontinen VK, et al. Adverse effects of perioperative paracetamol, NSAIDs, glucocorticoids, gabapentinoids and their combinations: a topical review. Acta Anaesthesiol Scand 2014;58(10):1182–98.

24. Krenzelok EP. The FDA Acetaminophen Advisory Committee Meeting - what is the future of acetaminophen in the United States? The perspective of a committee member. Clin Toxicol 2009;47(8):784–9.

25. Valentine AR, Carvalho B, Lazo TA, et al. Scheduled acetaminophen with as-needed opioids compared to as-needed acetaminophen plus opioids for post-cesarean pain management. Int J Obstet Anesth 2015;24(3):210–6.

26. Pavy TJ, Paech MJ, Evans SF. The effect of intravenous ketorolac on opioid requirement and pain after cesarean delivery. Anesth Analg 2001;92(4):1010–4.

27. Marret E, Kurdi O, Zufferey P, et al. Effects of nonsteroidal antiinflammatory drugs on patient-controlled analgesia morphine side effects: meta-analysis of randomized controlled trials. J Am Soc Anesthesiol 2005;102(6):1249–60.

28. Paech MJ, McDonnell NJ, Sinha A, et al. A randomised controlled trial of parecoxib, celecoxib and paracetamol as adjuncts to patient-controlled epidural analgesia after caesarean delivery. Anaesth Intensive Care 2014;42(1):15–22.

29. Ong C, Seymour R, Lirk P, et al. Combining paracetamol (acetaminophen) with nonsteroidal antiinflammatory drugs: a qualitative systematic review of analgesic efficacy for acute postoperative pain. Anesth Analg 2010;110:1170–9.

30. Tramer M, Williams J, Carroll D, et al. Comparing analgesic efficacy of nonsteroidal anti-inflammatory drugs given by different routes in acute and chronic pain: a qualitative systematic review. Acta Anaesthesiol Scand 1998;42:71–9.

31. Waldron NH, Jones CA, Gan TJ, et al. Impact of perioperative dexamethasone on postoperative analgesia and side-effects: systematic review and meta-analysis. Br J Anaesth 2013;110(2):191–200.

32. De Oliveira GS, Almeida MD, Benzon HT, et al. Perioperative single dose systemic dexamethasone for postoperative pain: a meta-analysis of randomized controlled trials. Anesthesiology 2011;115(3):575–88.

33. Cardoso MMS, Leite AO, Santos EA, et al. Effect of dexamethasone on prevention of postoperative nausea, vomiting and pain after caesarean section: a randomised, placebo-controlled, double-blind trial. Eur J Anaesthesiol 2013;30(3):102–5.

34. Ho K-Y, Gan TJ, Habib AS. Gabapentin and postoperative pain – a systematic review of randomized controlled trials. Pain 2006;126(1):91–101.

35. Tiippana EM, Hamunen K, Kontinen VK, et al. Do surgical patients benefit from perioperative gabapentin/pregabalin? A systematic review of efficacy and safety. Anesth Analg 2007;104(6):1545–56.

36. Moore A, Costello J, Wieczorek P, et al. Gabapentin improves postcesarean delivery pain management: a randomized, placebo-controlled trial. Anesth Analg 2011;112(1):167–73.

37. Short J, Downey K, Bernstein P, et al. A single preoperative dose of gabapentin does not improve postcesarean delivery pain management: a randomized, double-blind, placebo-controlled dose-finding trial. Anesth Analg 2012;115(6):1336–42.

38. Monks D, Hoppe D, Downey K, et al. A perioperative course of gabapentin does not produce a clinically meaningful improvement in analgesia after cesarean delivery: a randomized controlled trial. Anesthesiology 2015;123(2):320–6.

39. George RB, McKeen DM, Andreou P, et al. A randomized placebo-controlled trial of two doses of pregabalin for postoperative analgesia in patients undergoing abdominal hysterectomy. Can J Anesth 2014;61(6):551–7.

40. Zhang J, Ho KY, Wang Y. Efficacy of pregabalin in acute postoperative pain: a meta-analysis. Br J Anaesth 2011;106(4):454–62.

41. Engelman E, Cateloy F. Efficacy and safety of perioperative pregabalin for post-operative pain: a meta-analysis of randomized-controlled trials. Acta Anaesthesiol Scand 2011;55(8):927–43.

42. Kristensen JH, Ilett KF, Hackett LP, et al. Gabapentin and breastfeeding: a case report. J Hum Lact 2006;22(4):426–8.

43. Bell RF, Dahl JB, Moore R, et al. Peri-operative ketamine for acute post-operative pain: a quantitative and qualitative systematic review (Cochrane Review). Acta Anaesthesiol Scand 2005;49(10):1405–28.

44. Bauchat JR, Higgins N, Wojciechowski KG, et al. Low-dose ketamine with multi-modal postcesarean delivery analgesia: a randomized controlled trial. Int J Obstet Anesth 2011;20(1):3–9.

45. Rahmanian M, Leysi M, Hemmati AA, et al. The effect of low-dose intravenous ketamine on postoperative pain following cesarean section with spinal anesthesia: a randomized clinical trial. Oman Med J 2015;30(1):11–6.

46. Sen S, Ozmert G, Aydin ON, et al. The persisting analgesic effect of low-dose intravenous ketamine after spinal anaesthesia for Caesarean section. Eur J Anaesthesiol 2005;22(7):518–23.

47. Kashefi P. The benefits of intraoperative small-dose ketamine on postoperative pain after cesarean section. Anesthesiology 2006;104(4):27.

48. Snell P, Hicks C. An exploratory study in the UK of the effectiveness of three different pain management regimens for post-caesarean section women. Midwifery 2006;22:249–61.

49. Ruetzler K, Blome C, Nabecker S, et al. A randomised trial of oral versus intravenous opioids for treatment of pain after cardiac surgery. J Anesth 2014;28:580–6.

50. Madadi P, Moretti M, Djokanovic N, et al. Guidelines for maternal codeine use during breastfeeding. Can Fam Physician 2009;55(11):1077–8.

51. George J, Lin E, Hanna M, et al. The effect of intravenous opioid patient-controlled analgesia with and without background infusion on respiratory depression: a meta-analysis. J Opioid Manag 2010;6:47–54.

52. Hudcova J, McNicol E, Quah C, et al. Patient controlled opioid analgesia versus conventional opioid analgesia for postoperative pain. Cochrane Database Syst Rev 2006;(4):CD003348.

53. Bamigboye AA, Hofmeyr GJ. Local anaesthetic wound infiltration and abdominal nerves block during caesarean section for postoperative pain relief. Cochrane Database Syst Rev 2009;(3):CD006954.

54. Ventham NT, Hughes M, O'Neill S, et al. Systematic review and meta-analysis of continuous local anaesthetic wound infiltration versus epidural analgesia for postoperative pain following abdominal surgery. Br J Surg 2013;100(10):1280–9.

55. Lavand'homme P, Roelants F, Waterloos H, et al. Postoperative analgesic effects of continuous wound infiltration with diclofenac after elective cesarean delivery. Anesthesiology 2007;106:1220–5.

56. Eslamian L, Jalili Z, Jamal A, et al. Transversus abdominis plane block reduces postoperative pain intensity and analgesic consumption in elective cesarean delivery under general anesthesia. J Anesth 2012;26(3):334–8.

57. Liu S, Richman J, Thirlby R, et al. Efficacy of continuous wound catheters delivering local anesthetic for postoperative analgesia: a quantitative and qualitative

systematic review of randomized controlled trials. J Am Coll Surg 2006;203: 914–32.

58. Gupta A, Favaios S, Perniola A, et al. A meta-analysis of the efficacy of wound catheters for post-operative pain management. Acta Anaesthesiol Scand 2011; 55:785–96.

59. Zohar E, Shapiro A, Eidinov A, et al. Postcesarean analgesia: the efficacy of bupivacaine wound instillation with and without supplemental diclofenac. J Clin Anesth 2006;18(6):415–21.

60. Rackelboom T, Le Strat S, Silvera S, et al. Improving continuous wound infusion effectiveness for postoperative analgesia after cesarean delivery. Obs Gynaecol 2010;116:893–900.

61. Jabalameli M, Saryazdi H. The effect of subcutaneous dexamethasone added to bupivacaine on postcesarean pain: a randomized controlled trial. Ir J Med Sci 2010;35(1):21–6.

62. Kundra S, Singh RM, Singh G, et al. Efficacy of magnesium sulphate as an adjunct to ropivacaine in local infiltration for postoperative pain following lower segment caesarean section. J Clin Diagn Res 2016;10(4):UC18-22.

63. Carvalho B, Lemmens HJ, Ting V, et al. Postoperative subcutaneous instillation of low-dose ketorolac but not hydromorphone reduces wound exudate concentrations of interleukin-6 and interleukin-10 and improves analgesia following cesarean delivery. J Pain 2013;14(1):48–56.

64. Mishriky BM, George RB, Habib AS. Transversus abdominis plane block for analgesia after Cesarean delivery: a systematic review and meta-analysis. Can J Anesth 2012;59(8):766–78.

65. Abdallah FW, Halpern SH, Margarido CB. Transversus abdominis plane block for postoperative analgesia after Caesarean delivery performed under spinal anaesthesia? A systematic review and meta-analysis. Br J Anaesth 2012; 109(5):679–87.

66. Tan TT, Teoh WHL, Woo DCM, et al. A randomised trial of the analgesic efficacy of ultrasound-guided transversus abdominis plane block after caesarean delivery under general anaesthesia. Eur J Anaesthesiol 2012;29(2):88–94.

67. Chandon M, Bonnet A, Burg Y, et al. Ultrasound-guided transversus abdominis plane block versus continuous wound infusion for post-caesarean analgesia: a randomized trial. PLoS One 2014;9(8):e103971.

68. Aydogmus MT, Sinikoglu SN, Naki MM, et al. Comparison of analgesic efficiency between wound site infiltration and ultrasound-guided transversus abdominis plane block after cesarean delivery under spinal anaesthesia. Hippokratia 2014;18(1):28–31.

69. Telnes A, Skogvoll E, Lonnee H. Transversus abdominis plane block vs. wound infiltration in Caesarean section: a randomised controlled trial. Acta Anaesthesiol Scand 2015;59(4):496–504.

70. Støving K, Rothe C, Rosenstock CV, et al. Cutaneous sensory block area, muscle-relaxing effect, and block duration of the transversus abdominis plane block: a randomized, blinded, and placebo-controlled study in healthy volunteers. Reg Anesth Pain Med 2015;40(4):1–8.

71. Mirza F, Carvalho B. Transversus abdominis plane blocks for rescue analgesia following Cesarean delivery: a case series. Can J Anesth 2013;60(3):299–303.

72. Eslamian L, Kabiri-Nasab M, Agha-Husseini M, et al. Adding sufentanil to TAP block hyperbaric bupivacaine decreases post-cesarean delivery morphine consumption. Acta Med Iran 2016;54(3):185–90.

73. Wang LZ, Liu X, Zhang YF, et al. Addition of fentanyl to the ultrasound-guided transversus abdominis plane block does not improve analgesia following cesarean delivery. Exp Ther Med 2016;11(4):1441–6.

74. Bollag L, Richebe P, Siaulys M, et al. Effect of transversus abdominis plane block with and without clonidine on post-cesarean delivery wound hyperalgesia and pain. Reg Anesth Pain Med 2012;37(5):508–14.

75. Erdoğan Arı D, Yıldırım Ar A, Karadoğan F, et al. Ultrasound-guided transversus abdominis plane block in patients undergoing open inguinal hernia repair: 0.125% bupivacaine provides similar analgesic effect compared to 0.25% bupivacaine. J Clin Anesth 2016;28:41–6.

76. Griffiths JD, Le NV, Grant S, et al. Symptomatic local anaesthetic toxicity and plasma ropivacaine concentrations after transversus abdominis plane block for Caesarean section. Br J Anaesth 2013;110(6):996–1000.

77. Weiss E, Jolly C, Dumoulin J-L, et al. Convulsions in 2 patients after bilateral ultrasound-guided transversus abdominis plane blocks for cesarean analgesia. Reg Anesth Pain Med 2014;39(3):248–51.

78. Blanco R, Ansari T, Girgis E. Quadratus lumborum block for postoperative pain after caesarean section: a randomised controlled trial. Eur J Anaesthesiol 2015; 32(11):812–8.

79. Gasanova I, Alexander J, Ogunnaike B, et al. Transversus abdominis plane block versus surgical site infiltration for pain management after open total abdominal hysterectomy. Anesth Analg 2015;121(5):1383–8.

80. Simavli S, Kaygusuz I, Kinay T, et al. Bupivacaine-soaked absorbable gelatin sponges in cesarean section wounds: effect on postoperative pain, analgesic requirement, and hemodynamic profile. Int J Obs Anesth 2014;23(4):302–8.

81. Li Y, Dong Y. Preoperative music intervention for patients undergoing cesarean delivery. Int J Gynecol Obstet 2012;119(1):81–3.

82. Ebneshahidi A, Mohseni M. The effect of patient-selected music on early postoperative pain, anxiety, and hemodynamic profile in cesarean section surgery. J Altern Complement Med 2008;14(7):827–31.

83. Smith C, Guralnick M, Gelfand M, et al. The effects of transcutaneous electrical nerve stimulation on post-cesarean pain. Pain 1986;27:181–93.

84. Gillier CM, Sparks JR, Kriner R, et al. A randomized controlled trial of abdominal binders for the management of postoperative pain and distress after cesarean delivery. Int J Gynecol Obstet 2016;133(2):188–91.

85. Centers for Disease Control and Prevention. Progress in increasing breastfeeding and reducing racial/ethnic differences — United States, 2000-2008 births. MMWR 2013;62(05):77–80.

86. Montgomery A, Hale TW. ABM clinical protocol #15: analgesia and anesthesia for the breastfeeding mother, revised 2012. Breastfeed Med 2012;7(6):547–53.

87. Ilett K, Kristensen J. Drug use and breastfeeding. Expert Opin Drug Saf 2005; 4(4):745–68.

88. Spigset O, Hägg S. Analgesics and breast-feeding: safety considerations. Paediatr Drugs 2000;2(3):223–38.

89. American Academy of Pediatrics Committee on Drugs. The transfer of drugs and other chemicals into human milk. Pediatrics 2001;108(3):776–89.

90. Bond G, Holloway A. Anaesthesia and breast-feeding – the effect on mother and infant. Anaesth Intensive Care 1993;20(4):426–30.

91. Dalal PG, Bosak J, Berlin C. Safety of the breast-feeding infant after maternal anesthesia. Paediatr Anaesth 2014;24(4):359–71.

92. Gan TJ, Meyer TA, Apfel CC, et al. Society for ambulatory anesthesia guidelines for the management of postoperative nausea and vomiting. Anesth Analg 2007; 105:1615–28.

93. George R, Allen T, Habib A. Serotonin receptor antagonists for the prevention and treatment of pruritus, nausea, and vomiting in women undergoing cesarean delivery with intrathecal morphine: a systematic review and meta-analysis. Anesth Analg 2009;109(1):174–8.

94. Mishriky B, Habib A. Metoclopramide for nausea and vomiting prophylaxis during and after Caesarean delivery: a systematic review and meta-analysis. Br J Anaesth 2012;108(3):374–83.

95. Allen TK, Jones CA, Habib AS. Dexamethasone for the prophylaxis of postoperative nausea and vomiting associated with neuraxial morphine administration: a systematic review and meta-analysis. Anesth Analg 2012;114(4):813–22.

96. Habib AS, Reuveni J, Taguchi A, et al. A comparison of ondansetron with promethazine for treating postoperative nausea and vomiting in patients who received prophylaxis with ondansetron: a retrospective database analysis. Anesth Analg 2007;104(3):548–51.

97. Heffernan AM, Rowbotham DJ. Postoperative nausea and vomiting–time for balanced antiemesis? Br J Anaesth 2000;85(5):675–7.

98. Kjellberg F, Tramèr MR. Pharmacological control of opioid-induced pruritus: a quantitative systematic review of randomized trials. Eur J Anaesthesiol 2001; 18(6):346–57.

99. Bonnet M-P, Marret E, Josserand J, et al. Effect of prophylactic 5-HT3 receptor antagonists on pruritus induced by neuraxial opioids: a quantitative systematic review. Br J Anaesth 2008;101(3):311–9.

100. Wu Z, Kong M, Wang N, et al. Intravenous butorphanol administration reduces intrathecal morphine-induced pruritus after cesarean delivery: a randomized, double-blind, placebo-controlled study. J Anesth 2012;26(5):752–7.

101. Tamdee D, Charuluxananan S, Punjasawadwong Y, et al. A randomized controlled trial of pentazocine versus ondansetron for the treatment of intrathecal morphine-induced pruritus in patients undergoing cesarean delivery. Anesth Analg 2009;109(5):1606–11.

102. Siddik-Sayyid S, Aouad M, Taha S. Does ondansetron or granisetron prevent subarachnoid morphine-induced pruritus after cesarean delivery? Anesth Analg 2007;104(2):421–4.

103. Lockington PF, Fa'aea P. Subcutaneous naloxone for the prevention of intrathecal morphine induced pruritus in elective Caesarean delivery. Anaesthesia 2007;62(7):672–6.

104. Cohen SE, Ratner EF, Kreitzman TR, et al. Nalbuphine is better than naloxone for treatment of side effects after epidural morphine. Anesth Analg 1992;75(5): 747–52.

105. Cannesson M, Nargues N, Bryssine B, et al. Intrathecal morphine overdose during combined spinal-epidural block for Caesarean delivery. Br J Anaesth 2002; 89(6):925–7.

106. Abouleish E, Rawal N, Rashad MN. The addition of 0.2 mg subarachnoid morphine to hyperbaric bupivacaine for cesarean delivery: a prospective study of 856 cases. Reg Anesth 1991;16(3):137–40.

107. Practice guidelines for the prevention, detection, and management of respiratory depression associated with neuraxial opioid administration. Anesthesiology 2016;124(3):535–52.

108. Bloor M, Paech M. Nonsteroidal anti-inflammatory drugs during pregnancy and the initiation of lactation. Anesth Analg 2013;116(5):1063–75.
109. Wambach K. Drug therapy and breastfeeding. In: breastfeeding and human lactation. 5th edition. Burlington (MA): Jones & Bartlett Publishers; 2014. p. 171–206.
110. Hovinga CA, Pennell PB. Antiepileptic drug therapy in pregnancy II: fetal and neonatal exposure. Int Rev Neurobiol 2008;83:241–58.
111. Bloor M, Paech MJ, Kaye R. Tramadol in pregnancy and lactation. Int J Obstet Anesth 2012;21(2):163–7.

Should Nitrous Oxide Be Used for Laboring Patients?

Michael G. Richardson, MD[a],*, Brandon M. Lopez, MD[b],
Curtis L. Baysinger, MD[a]

KEYWORDS

- Nitrous oxide • Labor analgesia • Maternal satisfaction • Analgesic effectiveness
- Drug safety

KEY POINTS

- Unlike neuraxial labor analgesia, N_2O provides highly variable labor analgesia, ranging from very poor to very good.
- Despite this variability, parturients who choose to use N_2O where neuraxial analgesia is an option (including after trying N_2O) report satisfaction similar to that reported by women who use neuraxial analgesia. Parturients using N_2O report higher satisfaction than subsets of parturients who experience inadequate neuraxial labor analgesia.
- Regarding safety, parturient and neonatal adverse effects occur at rates similar to other techniques and may be no more frequent than in patients who undergo labor and delivery without analgesia. Environmental exposure and health risk to health care providers are minimal when proper scavenging of exhaled gas and adequate ventilation are used.
- Costs of administering N_2O appear similar to other alternatives for labor pain relief. Costs may be lower than for neuraxial techniques because non-anesthesia trained nursing staff can monitor nitrous oxide analgesia safely.
- N_2O analgesia provides a useful alternative for pain relief in parturients who decline neuraxial labor analgesia or who have contraindications to neuraxial blocks, and may offer advantages over patient-controlled systemic opioid administration and non-pharmacological techniques.

INTRODUCTION

Despite decades of widespread acceptance as a labor analgesic modality in numerous European countries, self-administered nitrous oxide (N_2O) has only

---

The authors have nothing to disclose.
[a] Department of Anesthesiology, Vanderbilt University Medical Center, 4202 VUH, 1211 Medical Center Drive, Nashville, TN 37232, USA; [b] Department of Anesthesiology, University of Florida College of Medicine, Gainesville, FL 32610, USA
* Corresponding author.
E-mail address: michael.g.richardson@vanderbilt.edu

Anesthesiology Clin 35 (2017) 125–143
http://dx.doi.org/10.1016/j.anclin.2016.09.011
1932-2275/17/© 2016 Elsevier Inc. All rights reserved.
anesthesiology.theclinics.com

recently captured great interest in the United States. The rare US medical center offering N_2O for labor in 2007[1] grew to an estimated 150 hospital labor and delivery units and 50 birthing centers in just a few years.[2] In contrast, roughly half of parturients in Finland, Norway, New South Wales Australia, Canada, and New Zealand and two-thirds of parturients in the United Kingdom and Sweden were estimated to have used N_2O when birthing centers were surveyed 10 years ago.[1] The availability of N_2O in institutions where neuraxial block is routine has been debated.[3,4] Despite a surprising paucity of evidence regarding its analgesic effectiveness, the long history and popularity of its use is compelling; the beneficial attributes of this modality are many, and the drawback are few (**Box 1**). The evidence as well as adverse effects, environmental exposure risks, and barriers and costs are reviewed, concluding that N_2O should be added to the modalities available to laboring parturients.

HISTORICAL CONSIDERATIONS

Several excellent reviews of the early history of N_2O use for anesthesia during surgery have been published,[5,6] and **Table 1** depicts a brief historical chronology. The discovery of N_2O is attributed to Joseph Priestly, who demonstrated its use in 1772.[5] In 1800, Humphry Davy reported that N_2O was useful at relieving toothache and associated it with pleasurable sensations during self-administration.[5] Dentist Horace Wells first suggested the use of N_2O as an anesthetic and self-administered it for a tooth removal; however, his public demonstration in Boston for surgery in 1845 was a failure.[5] William Morton, a year later in 1846, demonstrated the successful use of ether as an anesthetic at Massachusetts General Hospital, considered by some as the beginning of anesthesia as a medical practice.[7]

Other inhalational anesthetics preceded N_2O use in obstetrics. The year after ether for surgical anesthesia was successfully demonstrated in Boston, James Simpson successfully used it for a vaginal delivery in 1847[6]; however, wider acceptance of inhaled anesthesia for labor did not occur until John Snow administered chloroform to Queen Victoria during the birth of 2 children in 1853 and 1857.[6] The first use of N_2O in obstetrics is credited to Stanislav Klikovich, who developed a machine to deliver an 80/20 mixture of N_2O and oxygen.[8] Although he wrote of its safety and efficacy during labor in 1881, barriers, including cost, unfamiliarity of equipment, and access to equipment, prevented its widespread acceptance in laboring women.

During the early twentieth century, other devices for N_2O administration were developed. The Minnitt apparatus (A. Charles King, Ltd, London, England), introduced in 1933, delivered 50% N_2O in air. In 1936, the Royal College of Obstetricians and Gynecologists certified it as safe for use in obstetric patients attended by nurse midwives.[9] In 1961, Tunstall[10] described Entonox (BOC Healthcare, Manchester, England), a 50%/50% mix of N_2O and oxygen in a single cylinder, which was introduced into practice in the United Kingdom in 1965.[10] This combination was thought to be safer than mixing N_2O with air, and the device is currently in widespread use. Although N_2O was used in the United States during the 1970s, its use declined the following decade,[11] likely eclipsed by the growing popularity of neuraxial analgesia for labor during that time.

Although use of N_2O for surgical anesthesia has declined in the United States in the twenty-first century, the past 5 years have seen renewed interest in N_2O for labor.[12] In 2013, a barrier to N_2O use for labor in the United States was overcome with the

---

Box 1
Advantages and disadvantages for nitrous oxide analgesia

Advantages of N_2O

- Simplicity
  - Simple technique and equipment
  - Noninvasive technique
  - Self-administration method rapidly mastered by parturient

- Preservation of neurologic function
  - Sensory: able to experience the physical sensations of the childbirth process
  - Motor: strength and movement preserved
  - Autonomic: little hemodynamic effect; no respiratory depression

- Pharmacokinetics: rapid onset and offset of effects facilitated by low solubility

- Maternal control: able to titrate analgesia and balance desirable and undesirable effects according to her preferences

- Maternal distraction: distracting attention away from labor pain by focusing on breathing

- Easily discontinued in favor of switch to neuraxial analgesia, for the following reasons:
  - Ineffective N_2O analgesia as labor progresses and/or pain intensifies
  - Parturient fatigued/exhausted during long labor
  - Undesirable effects (sense of claustrophobia, physical and mental energy required to hold mask on face during each contraction)
  - Side effects (dysphoria, sedation, nausea)

- Allows for a low-risk trial, with option to switch to neuraxial modality

- Versatility
  - Supplement to inadequate or incomplete neuraxial analgesia
  - Quick option when delivery is imminent, too late for neuraxial
  - Supplement to local infiltration and/or pudendal block for repair of perineal lacerations/ birth trauma

- Often effective for milder pain: relative lesser analgesic effectiveness may be adequate for
  - Early labor, milder labor pain
  - Parturient using effective coping skills

- Additional option: for women who desire neuraxial analgesia but who have contraindications to it

Disadvantages of N_2O

- Incomplete analgesia: significantly less effective in treating labor pain than neuraxial techniques

- Side effects
  - Nausea
  - Dizziness/dysphoria/sedation
  - Sense of claustrophobia

- Requires active participation

---

commercial reintroduction of an N_2O apparatus (Porter Nitronox, Porter Instrument, Parker Hannifin, Hatfield, PA, USA).[13] This small, easy-to-use, self-contained device (**Fig. 1**) is marketed to hospitals, academic medical institutions, and birthing centers as an alternative to natural or neuraxial analgesia for laboring parturients. Advantages of the Nitronox apparatus over the Entonox system include use of readily available N_2O and oxygen E-cylinders (not a proprietary N_2O-oxygen cylinder) and the capability of gas scavenging.

Table 1
History of nitrous oxide and other inhalational anesthetic administration

Date:	Event
1772	Joseph Priestly synthesized N_2O.
1800	Humphry Davy described N_2O use to relieve pain.
1845	Horace Wells demonstrated use of N_2O for surgery.
1847	James Simpson used ether for vaginal delivery.
1853	John Snow used chloroform for Queen Victoria's labor.
1881	Stanislav Klikovich published the first study of N_2O use in laboring women.
1934	Minnitt apparatus for N_2O self-administration was introduced.
1961	Tunstall introduced the Entonox, combining N_2O with oxygen in one cylinder.
2013	Nitronox machine becomes widely available in the United States.
2015	More than 20 hospital systems and 30 birthing centers in the United States report offering N_2O for labor analgesia.

NITROUS OXIDE PHARMACOKINETICS AND PHARMACODYNAMICS

N_2O is a vapor anesthetic that is tasteless and odorless. It is a weak anesthetic agent with a minimum alveolar concentration more than 100% at 1 atm, which confers safety during administration of the 50% concentration. N_2O has very low blood/gas solubility,

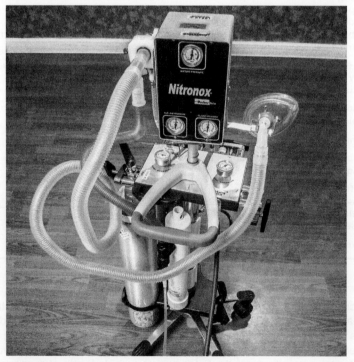

Fig. 1. N_2O apparatus. Photograph shows disposable circuitry and mask, N_2O tank, mixing box allowing delivery of only a 50% N_2O mixture, with wall source oxygen and scavenging tubing. (*Courtesy of* Porter Instrument, Parker Hannifin, Hatfield, PA; with permission.)

and Waud and Waud[14] showed that peak brain concentrations occurred 60 seconds after onset of its administration in laboring patients. Its mechanism of action, however, is not well understood. Maze and Fuginaga[15] hypothesized that N_2O induces release of endogenous opioid peptides in the periaqueductal gray area of the midbrain. These peptides stimulate descending noradrenergic neuronal pathways, which modulate pain processing by alpha-2 receptors in the dorsal horn of the spinal cord.[15] Gruss and colleagues[16] showed that N_2O has poor action at γ-aminobutyric acid receptors like other volatile anesthetics but noted that N-methyl-D-aspartate (NMDA) receptor inhibition is the mechanism most likely responsible for its anesthetic effects. Richebé and colleagues[17] demonstrated that the NMDA antagonist properties of N_2O prevented enhancement of pain sensitivity and reduced postoperative pain. The release of endogenous opioids and the inhibition of NMDA receptors are likely responsible for the analgesic effects of N_2O.

NITROUS OXIDE: VARIABLE ANALGESIC EFFECTIVENESS

Despite its introduction as a labor analgesic nearly 6 decades ago, its subsequent routine use throughout Europe, and its growing popularity in the United States, evidence regarding the effectiveness of N_2O is surprisingly limited. A 2002 systematic review with strict criteria for inclusion (randomization, adequate control group, effectiveness assessments by parturients at the time of or shortly after intervention) identified only 11 trials of adequate quality for review. Data on 340 parturients were analyzed from the studies, which were conducted between 1961 and 1995 (7 before 1985).[18] Drawing conclusions regarding analgesic effectiveness was difficult as the concentration of N_2O studied was variable (30%–70%), as were methods of administration, methods and timing of effectiveness assessments, and comparator modalities (many now outmoded, such as repeated doses of intramuscular meperidine, inhalational methoxyflurane, anesthesiologist administered enflurane, transcutaneous electrical nerve stimulation, and so forth). A systematic review 12 years later added little.[19] It identified 12 randomized controlled trials examining effectiveness, including 9 of the same trials as the prior review, excluded 2 low-quality studies from the prior review,[20,21] and added only a single new study.[22] Both reviews deemed the strength of evidence for N_2O labor analgesia effectiveness to be insufficient to make conclusions, owing primarily to unsatisfactory study design.[18,19] However, N_2O is an alternative analgesic option for some women.

Although neuraxial techniques are more effective overall in providing labor pain relief than N_2O, most studies identify subsets of women who report significant analgesic effectiveness from N_2O, with many stating that they would choose it again for a future delivery.[21,23–30] Unlike the consistently reliable effectiveness of neuraxial analgesia, N_2O yields variable analgesic effectiveness. In a postpartum survey study of 1096 nulliparous and 1386 parous Swedish women, most (84% and 72%, respectively) rated epidural analgesia as very effective. Despite N_2O being less effective, 38% of nulliparous and 49% of parous women also reported N_2O to be *very* effective.[23] In another study, more than 800 Finnish parturients were assessed before and after various labor analgesic interventions, including N_2O, epidural alone, and epidural or paracervical block after trying various modalities (N_2O, meperidine, water blocks).[24] Although epidural analgesia was superior to all other modalities during the first stage of labor, and a subset of women using N_2O subsequently switched to regional blocks, many women chose to continue with N_2O alone for the entirety of their labor, despite the availability of alternatives. After delivery, 94% of women who used epidural analgesia reported good analgesic effectiveness. In contrast, 28% of those who delivered with

N_2O alone reported poor and 39% moderate analgesic adequacy, yet 33% rated analgesia as good. Holdcroft and Morgan[25] conducted an observational study of 663 parturients who delivered vaginally using N_2O, meperidine, or both. Of the 130 who used N_2O alone, 31% reported no pain relief, 18% slight, yet 47% reported satisfactory and 4% complete analgesia. Most recently, Dammer and colleagues[26] reported on 66 laboring women who chose to use N_2O soon after introduction of an inhaled N_2O analgesia program in a German academic center. Reasons for choosing N_2O included refusal to use epidural analgesia (59%), inability to place an epidural (23%), inadequate epidural analgesia (8%), or unspecified reasons (11%). Analgesic effectiveness was variable. Two-thirds of women reported being *quite* or *very likely* to use N_2O again for labor, and one-third reported *absolutely not, a little,* or *moderately likely.*

In summary, wide ranges in analgesic effectiveness are consistently reported in published studies. Factors that predict N_2O effectiveness as a sole analgesic agent have yet to be determined. However, it is clear that N_2O serves as an effective analgesic modality for some women who choose to use it.

WHAT MATTERS: EFFECTIVE PAIN RELIEF VERSUS SATISFACTION?

Although effectiveness of pain relief is a primary determinant in many parturients' reported satisfaction with labor analgesic care, especially with neuraxial modalities,[24,31–36] it is clearly not the only factor.[34,37–40] Among 28 women with a priori plans to use labor epidural analgesia, effective pain relief (confidence in timely access to it and analgesic effectiveness) was viewed as beneficial in regaining self-control and ability to focus, think, and participate in the birth process.[34] Of note, parturients also identified other factors important to birth experience satisfaction, such as preservation of bodily sensations of labor, mobility, and strength. This study highlighted the multidimensional nature of the parturients' experience of labor analgesia, including measures of cognitive, emotional, and physical domains. Consistent with this, a systematic review of 137 reports investigating factors influencing parturients' assessments of their childbirth experiences identified factors that strongly affect parturient satisfaction with the childbirth experience, including personal expectations, caregiver support, quality of the relationship with her caregiver, and involvement in decision-making.[37] The development and implementation of coping-with-pain algorithms may be an alternative to numerical pain rating scales that quantify only labor pain.[38,39] The experience of labor is unique to each individual and comprises the complex interplay between physical, physiologic, psychological, emotional, social, and cultural dimensions.[38,39] Unlike traumatic, postoperative, or other pathologic pain, the pain of labor accompanies the unique process of giving birth to new life. The coping algorithm approach does not eliminate but rather de-emphasizes pain as the dominant or sole dimension of the labor experience and allows for a more holistic or global patient-centered assessment. If the parturient is coping well, then continued support is given. If not, then various dimensions can be assessed and appropriate interventions suggested or offered.[39] Finally, a qualitative content analysis of 2005 national survey data from 1573 US parturients who delivered a singleton baby revealed the high importance of timely and effective neuraxial analgesia for those who requested it.[40] However, analgesia was one among many other factors identified by women who were asked open-ended questions about the best and worst aspects of their birth experience.

In summary, although effectiveness of pain relief heavily influences satisfaction with labor analgesia for many women, especially with for those who choose neuraxial modalities, it is not the sole determinant. This may explain the consistent popularity of

N$_2$O labor analgesia use in Europe, and its growing popularity in the United States. Many parturients who deliver with N$_2$O, in spite of having ready access to neuraxial modalities, report high satisfaction despite incomplete analgesia.

NITROUS OXIDE: 5-YEAR EXPERIENCE AT A HIGH-RISK ACADEMIC CENTER

N$_2$O has been offered as an option for all laboring women at Vanderbilt Medical Center since June 2011. Soon after admission, anesthesiology personnel assess every woman with a viable pregnancy and counsel them regarding neuraxial and N$_2$O analgesic options provided by the obstetric anesthesiology service, including benefits, side effects, risks, limitations on mobility, and the relative level of analgesia that may be expected. Consistently, one in 5 laboring women selects N$_2$O analgesia during some point during labor (**Fig. 2**). Of those who do and deliver vaginally, 60% use N$_2$O as the sole analgesic, whereas 40% switch to neuraxial analgesia (see **Fig. 2**). In contrast, of those who start with N$_2$O and ultimately deliver by cesarean, the conversion rate during labor is higher, 63%, possibly due to longer and more painful labor associated with those whose labor course culminates in cesarean delivery.[41,42] Reasons for converting to neuraxial analgesia after N$_2$O include the following:

- *Inadequate analgesia*: Some women switch to neuraxial analgesia because they experience little or no analgesic effect soon after trying N$_2$O. Others are satisfied with N$_2$O analgesia initially but convert later, as contraction pain intensifies, whether because of progress of labor or oxytocin augmentation.

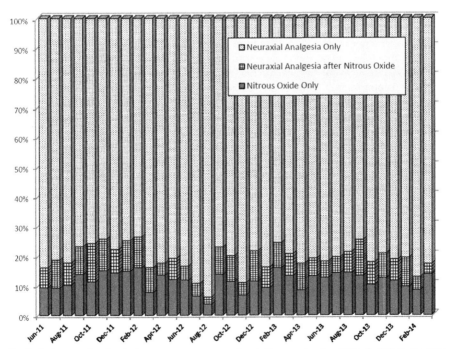

Fig. 2. Labor analgesia choices among women who deliver vaginally at Vanderbilt University Medical Center. Image shows monthly labor analgesic usage pattern for neuraxial analgesia, N$_2$O analgesia only, and conversion to neuraxial analgesia after using N$_2$O over a 34-month period.

- *Undesirable side effects:* These side effects include dizziness, nausea, sedation, and a sense of claustrophobia from the mask.
- *Fatigue/exhaustion:* N_2O use requires being awake and actively holding the mask to the face. As labor pain intensifies or during lengthy labors, some women tire of the effort and coordination required to self-administer the drug. During lengthy labors and/or when parturients are exhausted or sleep deprived, some women opt for the rest and sleep conferred by the complete analgesia produced by neuraxial modalities.

Analysis of routine postpartum assessments of analgesic effectiveness and satisfaction among 6242 parturients who delivered vaginally during a 34-month period (2011–2014) revealed variable levels of effectiveness (21% poor, 27% intermediate, 52% high) among the 678 women who delivered with N_2O alone, yet satisfaction among these women was as high as and not different from those who used neuraxial analgesia (n = 5103) or those who chose neuraxial analgesia after first using N_2O (n = 461).[43] This observation may be due to differences in expected analgesic effects of N_2O versus neuraxial analgesia.[36]

In summary, N_2O seems to serve the analgesic needs of the subset of laboring women who choose to use it, including women whose birth plans include limited medication, unencumbered movement, strong preference to avoid neuraxial techniques, and a high level of control. Some parturients seek to deliver at the authors' institution specifically because they offer N_2O for labor. Additionally, N_2O serves as an alternative when there are contraindications to neuraxial blocks (eg, coagulation disorders, spine abnormalities, or prior spine surgery).

NITROUS OXIDE ANALGESIA VERSUS OTHER NON-NEURAXIAL TECHNIQUES

Unfortunately, there is no useful evidence comparing N_2O with other non-neuraxial analgesic modalities or nonpharmacologic interventions. Most studies of such alternative interventions reveal modest or no analgesic effectiveness, including maternal childbirth preparation,[44] relaxation techniques,[45] water immersion/whirlpool therapy,[46] acupuncture/acupressure,[47] transcutaneous nerve stimulation (TENS),[48] and subcutaneous water injection.[49] A single observational study examined pain relief and satisfaction from use of TENS, N_2O, intramuscular meperidine, and epidural analgesia.[31] Most women reported some pain relief from TENS and N_2O, and half reported no relief from intramuscular opioid.

Similarly, comparisons of N_2O with systemic opioid analgesics are sparse. Analgesia produced by intramuscular opioids is reported to be modest[50] or ineffective (active advanced labor).[51] Intravenous administration seems to improve effectiveness compared with the intramuscular route, especially if patient-controlled modalities are used.[52] Patient-controlled intravenous remifentanil has advantages of rapid onset of action and peak effect compared with other opioids, which may allow timing of administration to coincide with uterine contraction pain.[52] Unfortunately, significant maternal oxygen desaturation,[53] nausea,[54] and pruritus[52] are common. A single study comparing N_2O and patient-controlled intravenous remifentanil demonstrated slightly greater analgesic effectiveness but greater sedation with remifentanil.[55] No hypoxemic episodes were observed in the remifentanil group, although supplemental oxygen was administered to mothers. Without supplemental oxygen, oxygen desaturation was observed in 25% of parturients using remifentanil.[56] The implication for increased monitoring, perhaps requiring one-to-one nursing,[53] is a drawback of remifentanil analgesia.

In summary, evidence comparing N_2O with non-neuraxial pharmacologic or nonpharmacologic alternatives is lacking. Systemic opioid administration is the only other modality that has been demonstrated to produce effective analgesia in some women but has more drawbacks compared with N_2O.

ADVERSE MATERNAL AND NEONATAL EFFECTS

N_2O is generally well tolerated, without major side effects. Some of the reported adverse reactions and contraindications to N_2O for labor are presented in **Box 2**. Although N_2O likely has little direct effect on ventilatory drive, its use during labor has been associated with brief self-limited maternal oxygen desaturations between labor contractions.[57] Self-administration techniques involve focused inhalation of the gas to obtain analgesic effects. Hyperventilation during uterine contractions, and associated hypocapnia, may be the cause of occasional oxygen desaturation.[58] The alternative hypothesis, diffusion hypoxemia during room air breathing between contractions, is an unlikely cause.[58] Of note, oxygen desaturation is observed during some unmedicated labors.[59]

A small subset of women experience nausea when using N_2O. In a large systemic review of multiple studies by Likis and colleagues,[19] nausea was reported to occur at rates ranging from 0% to 45%. The possibility of increased nausea with the use of N_2O should be discussed with the parturient, especially if she is already nauseous from labor. Likis and colleagues'[19] review also reported an incidence of dizziness that ranged from 3% to 23%. Dizziness is typically well tolerated if the parturient is informed, but it sometimes requires discontinuation of its use. In a another study of 1000 laboring women, 4% of parturients reported drowsiness, 18% experienced reduced awareness, and 5% exhibited mask phobia.[60] Unconsciousness is most probably rare; 2 studies by Arthurs and Rosen[61] and Westling and colleagues[62] found a 0% incidence. Adding systemic opioids to N_2O analgesia (and epidural analgesia) may increase the incidence of maternal respiratory depression and intermittent hypoxemia.[59] The discontinuation of opioids, such as butorphanol, is recommended 2 hours

---

Box 2
Maternal side effects of nitrous oxide administration: contraindications to use

Maternal side effects

- Nausea and vomiting

- Dizziness

- Drowsiness

- Respiratory depression

- Unconsciousness

Contraindications

- Absolute
  - Recent pneumothorax
  - Recent retinal surgery
  - Recent middle ear or sinus infection
  - Known vitamin B12 deficiency

- Relative
  - Pernicious anemia
  - Extensive bowel resection due to Crohn disease
  - Vegans who do not consume legumes
  - Methionine synthetase deficiency or reduction

before initiating N_2O. In summary, the incidence of various maternal side effects attributable to N_2O administration alone is difficult to determine given the lack of adequate comparative studies.

Significant adverse effects on the neonate have not been reported. In an obstetric outcome study conducted in the United Kingdom, the Medical Research Council noted no serious neonatal effects that could be attributed to N_2O administration.[63] Likis and colleagues[19] reviewed 29 studies reporting fetal or neonatal adverse outcomes, specifically umbilical cord blood gases and Apgar scores, and reported no significant differences between mothers using N_2O compared with other labor pain methods or no analgesia. Leong and colleagues[32] observed no differences in fetal outcomes at 1 and 5 minutes after delivery between groups receiving N_2O with meperidine or epidural analgesia, and no newborn had an Apgar score lower than 7 at 5 minutes. Stefani and colleagues[64] conducted validated neurobehavioral assessments on infants at 15 minutes, 2 hours, and 24 hours of age and showed no significant differences between neonates born to mothers receiving 30% to 50% N_2O or no inhalational agent during the second stage of labor. Although there is no evidence of adverse effects of N_2O for the fetus, the strength of that evidence is far from conclusive; much remains unknown about the effects on the developing brain.[65] Concerns regarding the neurotoxic effects of N_2O (and other anesthetic agents) on the developing brain have been raised because of studies showing neuroapoptosis in rodents exposed to anesthetic agents in large doses.[66] Most studies involve concentrations and durations of agent exposure far greater than typically used during general anesthesia.[67]

CONTRAINDICATIONS

Contraindications to N_2O use in laboring patients are few (see **Box 2**). The potential for N_2O to expand closed gas spaces is well known; caution is advised in women who have had a recent pneumothorax, pneumocephalus, venous air embolism, bowel obstruction, retinal surgery, middle ear surgery, or sinus infections.[68] N_2O should also be avoided in patients with known pulmonary hypertension and certain congenital heart diseases because of its known effects on pulmonary vascular resistance. Risks of N_2O use in the presence of reduced methionine synthetase activity have been debated.[13] Although no adverse effects have been reported in laboring parturients, caution is advised in women with B12 deficiency (methylenetetrahydrofolate reductase; megaloblastic anemia) owing to rare reports of subacute combined degeneration in severely vitamin B12–deficient patients with prolonged exposure to high concentrations of N_2O during general anesthesia.[69]

HEALTH CARE WORKER EXPOSURE, ENVIRONMENTAL, EQUIPMENT, AND ADMINISTRATIVE CONCERNS

Although inhaled N_2O offers an alternative to neuraxial analgesia and has advantages compared with other non-neuraxial alternatives, several practical issues must be considered before introducing a N_2O program (**Box 3**).

HEALTH CARE WORKER EXPOSURE

The National Institute for Occupational Safety and Health (NIOSH) sets an exposure limit of 25 ppm as a time weighted average (TWA) during periods of anesthetic administration.[70] This recommendation, set in 1977 and not reviewed since 1994, was not intended to prevent long-term health consequences for workers but rather to prevent

---

Box 3
Health care worker exposure, environmental, equipment, and administrative concerns

Health care worker exposure

- Government-established exposure limits are measured as time weighted averages and vary by country.

- Exposure limits may be exceeded for staff with prolonged close contact with parturients using N_2O.

- Correct apparatus use by patients, effective scavenging systems, and room ventilation reduce exposure to acceptable levels.

Exposure and health safety

- N_2O exposure does not seem to increase health care worker risks, except slightly reduced fecundity among women with prolonged exposure to high N_2O levels.

Environmental effects

- The greenhouse gas potency of N_2O is 300 times greater than carbon dioxide, but the overall contribution of medical N_2O to atmospheric warming is miniscule.

Administrative procedures and clinical use

- Policies that govern N_2O administration must comply with institutional sedation and analgesia policies as outlined by the institution's department of anesthesia.

- Effective obstetric and patient instruction is needed for effective use.

- Safe administration can be monitored by nonanesthesia personnel.

- Cost of administration is comparable with neuraxial techniques; personnel costs may be lower if nonanesthesia personnel conduct administration.

---

possible effects of exposure on health providers' sight and audio acuity and mental performance. NIOSH based their 25 ppm recommendation on decreased audiovisual performance noted when test subjects were exposed to 50 ppm N_2O.[71] The levels of N_2O exposure sufficient to pose health risks to obstetric providers are unknown. A meta-analysis of 16 studies published before 2002 failed to establish an association between occupational exposure and risk and concluded that evidence to date could not serve to set occupational health standards for exposure.[18] This finding is reflected in the wide range of exposure limits in various countries: France, United States, 25 ppm; Italy, Belgium 50 ppm; Sweden, United Kingdom, 100 ppm; Germany, 200 ppm (duration up to 15 minutes, 4 times per day).[72]

Levels commonly exceed 25 ppm when N_2O is administered without effective scavenging. Such levels of exposure are also more likely to occur in labor and delivery facilities with minimal room ventilation.[73–76] Mills and colleagues[73] measured environmental N_2O exposure among nurse midwives during N_2O use in labor and delivery units where it was not scavenged and delivery rooms were not ventilated. Personal N_2O samplers worn close to the face are used to measure average ambient N_2O levels in parts per million for each shift. Median N_2O exposure during 242 sampling periods was 23 ppm, with a range of 0 to 1638 ppm. In 23% of samples, mean levels exceeded 100 ppm during a shift, with 7 (3%) measuring more than 500 ppm. This finding compared with median N_2O levels of 12 ppm in 111 shifts where midwives had not worked with Entonox.

Routine scavenging and labor room ventilation effectively reduces staff exposure considerably. Munley and colleagues[74] reported 2.5-fold reductions in measured

N_2O exposure when a rudimentary scavenging system was introduced during N_2O use. Chessor and colleagues[75] compared conventional scavenging with a novel mask scavenging system similar to that commonly used now in the United States and noted reductions in nurse exposure from 69 ppm to 40 ppm. The greatest reduction in ambient N_2O levels is achieved when effective N_2O scavenging is combined with room ventilation. The use of a scavenging system similar to the system used with Nitronox equipment currently in use in the United States yielded 8-hour TWA levels of 7.5 to 21.0 ppm in ventilated labor and delivery rooms.[76] Brief periods of high peak exposure were few. N_2O levels, ranging from 50 to 110 ppm, of 15-minute duration, were measured 8 times in 11 of 15 midwives during 88 total hours of sampling. Room air monitoring on the labor and delivery suite at Vanderbilt Medical Center has failed to detect N_2O concentrations in excess of 25 ppm, and obstetric nurse exposure measured by badge dosimeters have not exceeded NIOSH TWA limits.

In summary, equipment that includes N_2O demand valves and effective scavenging systems when used in ventilated delivery rooms seems to limit obstetric health care provider exposure to levels that do not significantly exceed governmental standards.

NITROUS OXIDE EXPOSURE AND HEALTH SAFETY RISK

Survey studies linking N_2O exposure to health care worker reproductive hazards appeared in the 1960s and 1970s. Study subjects were either operating room personnel or dental assistants, and all were exposed to levels of N_2O and other anesthetic gases that far exceeded that found in any current health care environment. Despite such high exposure levels, these studies reported marginal statistical significance for increased risk (relative risk for spontaneous abortion, 1.3; congenital anomalies, 1.2), which may be explained by confounding variables (eg, survey bias, reporting bias, or other uncontrolled variables).[77,78] One study of dental assistants reported statistically significant lower fertility among a small subset of women exposed to very high levels of N_2O (5 or more hours of exposure per week in an unscavenged environment),[79] levels not achieved in contemporary operating rooms or labor and delivery environments. The failure to observe increased rates of congenital anomalies among women who have received N_2O during surgery in the first 2 trimesters of pregnancy or during cervical cerclage placement is reassuring.[72] Two studies examining reproductive outcomes among Swedish midwives exposed to N_2O failed to reveal an increased risk of spontaneous abortion among those exposed to N_2O.[80,81] Overall, current epidemiologic data do not support increased reproductive health risks among health care workers exposed to subanesthetic concentrations of N_2O during care of laboring women but slightly reduced fecundity among women with very high levels of exposure may occur.[80]

ENVIRONMENTAL CONCERNS

N_2O is a potent greenhouse gas, approximately 300 times more potent at trapping atmospheric heat than carbon dioxide; most N_2O administered for anesthetic purposes ultimately ends up in the atmosphere.[82] However, medical use has been estimated to contribute to less than 0.05% of total atmospheric warming and is responsible for less than 1.0% of all N_2O in the atmosphere.[82] Swedish manufacturers have developed equipment that reclaims and destroys N_2O. Ek and Tjus[83] recently reported a near halving of emissions countrywide from 2002 to 2010, thanks to the widespread use of these units in Sweden. The medical use of N_2O has little environmental impact.

ADMINISTRATIVE PROCEDURES AND CLINICAL USE

N_2O administration should comply with the anesthesia and sedation policies unique to each institution. Within the United States, these policies should follow the Conditions of Participation (42 CFR 482.52) recently updated by the Centers for Medicare and Medicaid Services, which direct that the department of anesthesia at each facility develop and implement all policies for sedation and analgesia. Current American Society of Anesthesiologists' practice guidelines for sedation and analgesia categorize patient self-administered 50% N_2O as analgesia or minimal sedation,[84] so administration and monitoring by an anesthesia provider are not required. The United Kingdom has a long history of safe provision by nonanesthesia personnel of self-administered N_2O to laboring women. Monitoring parturients with pulse oximetry within 2 hours of having received systemic narcotics is recommended.[85] Policies for monitoring by nursing staff should be delineated. One-on-one nursing care is not necessary, in contrast to recommendations for one-on-one nursing care when patient-controlled intravenous opioid analgesia is used for labor analgesia.[53,86] Staff training has been reported to be effective in training such nonanesthesia providers for safe use.[87]

Effective N_2O labor analgesia requires proper patient use; this is best achieved by providing the parturient with good instruction, coaching, and initial supervision/monitoring to ensure proper use and confirm clinical effect. The combination of a low blood-gas solubility coefficient and use of a high (50%) inspired concentration, promotes rapid N_2O uptake. This rapid uptake accelerates onset analgesic effects but also prevents alveolar concentrations from approaching the inspired concentration during the typical intermittent use during uterine contractions. Ideally, patients should begin intermittent use 30 to 45 seconds before peak contraction strength and take 4 to 5 consecutive breaths.[88] If uterine contractions are regular in period, then analgesia could begin before onset of a contraction is sensed. **Table 2** outlines a recommended technique for administration.

Table 2
Nitrous oxide analgesia: technique and patient instruction

Steps	Action
Assess parturient	Identify potential contraindications (see **Box 2**) Full discussion of benefits, limitations, side effects (dizziness, nausea) Confirm that parturient can self-administer using mask apparatus Determine if patients learn the technique while laboring
Prepare for administration	Inspect equipment before administration Provide patient instruction Hold mask to face, with complete seal to ensure effective drug administration Timing strategy: Initiate inhalation anticipating onset of contraction (if labor is regular) or as soon as contraction is sensed (if labor is irregular)
Monitor mother during use and provide feedback on technique	Confirm complete seal between face and mask during inspiration (drug uptake) and exhalation (ensure effective scavenging) Assess and record initial vital signs and oxygen saturation at beginning of use Assess for effectiveness and satisfaction; if not effective or dissatisfaction, remind parturient of alternative options Assess for and manage side effects (sedation, nausea)

EQUIPMENT

The N_2O labor analgesia apparatus may include a single gas cylinder containing a one-to-one mix of N_2O and oxygen supplied at 2000 psi (both in gas phase, owing to the Poynting effect), most often used in Europe (eg, Entonox). In the United States, the apparatus most commonly draws the gases from separate sources (N_2O from an attached E cylinder and oxygen from a wall source or E cylinder) to provide a one-to-one ratio output. On a practical note, N_2O remains in a liquid phase inside a compressed gas cylinder, so long as the gas phase remains at 745 psi. Once the liquid is depleted, cylinder pressure decreases precipitously. If a parturient who was experiencing satisfactory analgesia develops a sudden increase in pain, an empty N_2O cylinder should be considered.

All devices should use a disposable circuit attached to a mask and demand valve that delivers N_2O only during negative pressure generated by patient inhalation. The demand valve limits N_2O flow only to those times when patients are actively inhaling (see **Fig. 1**). A scavenger device attached to the mask/demand valve assembly is essential to remove exhaled gas and minimize environmental contamination. Nearly 70% of exhaled N_2O can be captured with such systems.[86] Finally, despite lack of reported instances, N_2O, as with other anesthetic agents, has abuse potential, either by health care workers or persons other than the patients to whom it is prescribed. Equipment should be stored in secure areas when not in use, and the institution's substance abuse policy should apply.

COST

Several investigators[89] have noted that N_2O administration is inexpensive, although specific costs of providing care have not been published. Disposable supply costs are similar to those for neuraxial blocks (approximately $20 hospital cost at Vanderbilt), and capital costs are not prohibitive (approximately $5000 per apparatus). The equipment is robust and has a long life expectancy.[89] Personnel costs are probably lower than those involving neuraxial blockades if N_2O is administered by nurse midwives or labor and delivery nursing personnel, reflecting differences in labor costs versus that of anesthesia-trained persons. The cost-effectiveness of N_2O analgesia needs further investigation.[90]

SUMMARY

Each parturient has personal preferences and needs, which are shaped by the uniqueness of her life experience. Furthermore, these preferences and needs are dynamic and often change during the course of her labor. Although N_2O is less effective in treating labor pain than neuraxial analgesic modalities, it has consistently served the needs and preferences of a small but significant subset of parturients. Including N_2O in the repertoire of modalities that obstetric anesthesiologists offer to alleviate pain and suffering, and to facilitate effective coping and maternal satisfaction, is consistent with a commitment to addressing the needs of all parturients.

REFERENCES

1. Rooks JP. Nitrous oxide for pain in labor-why not in the United States? Birth 2007; 34:3–5.
2. Collins M. Top ten misconceptions about the use of nitrous oxide in labor. AWHONN Connections August 14, 2015. Available at: https://awhonnconnections.org/2015/08/14/top-ten-misconceptions-about-the-use-of-nitrous-oxide-in-labor/. Accessed May 15, 2016.

3. Yentis SM. The use of Entonox® for labour pain should be abandoned. Proposer. Int J Obstet Anesth 2001;10:25–7.
4. Clyburn P. The use of Entonox® for labour pain should be abandoned. Int J Obstet Anesth 2001;10:27–9.
5. Frost EA. A history of nitrous oxide. In: Eger EI, editor. Nitrous oxide/N20. New York: Elsevier; 1985. p. 1–22.
6. Caton D. What a blessing she had chloroform: the medical and social response to the pain of childbirth 1800 – present. New Haven (CO): Yale University Press; 1999.
7. Cartwright FF. The English pioneers of anaesthesia. Bristol (United Kingdom): John Wright and Sons Ltd; 1952.
8. Richards W, Parbrook G, Wilson J. Stanislav Klikovitch (1853-1910). Pioneer of nitrous oxide and oxygen analgesia. Anaesthesia 1976;31:933–40.
9. O'Sullivan EP. Dr. Robert James Minnitt 1889-1974: a pioneer of inhalational analgesia. J R Soc Med 1989;82:221–2.
10. Tunstall ME. Obstetric analgesia. The use of a fixed nitrous oxide and oxygen mixture from one cylinder. Lancet 1961;2:964.
11. Hawkins J, Gibbs C, Orleans M, et al. Obstetric anesthesia work force survey, 1981 versus 1992. Anesthesiology 1997;87:135–43.
12. Brown SM, Sneyd JR. Nitrous oxide in modern anaesthetic practice. BJA Educ 2016;16:87–91.
13. Starr SA, Baysinger CL. Inhaled nitrous oxide for labor analgesia. Anesthesiol Clin 2013;31:623–34.
14. Waud BE, Waud DR. Calculated kinetics of distribution of nitrous oxide and methoxyflurane during intermittent administration in obstetrics. Anesthesiology 1970;32:306–16.
15. Maze M, Fuginaga M. Recent advances in understanding the actions and toxicity of nitrous oxide. Anaesthesia 2000;55:311–4.
16. Gruss M, Bushell TJ, Bright DP, et al. Two-pore-domain K+ channels are a novel target for the anesthetic gases xenon, nitrous oxide, and cyclopropane. Mol Pharmacol 2004;65:443–52.
17. Richebé P, Rivat C, Creton C, et al. Nitrous oxide revisited: evidence for potent antihyperalgesic properties. Anesthesiology 2005;103:845–54.
18. Rosen MA. Nitrous oxide for relief of labor pain. A systematic review. Am J Obstet Gynecol 2002;186:S110–26.
19. Likis FE, Andrews JC, Collins MR, et al. Nitrous oxide for the management of labor pain: a systematic review. Anesth Analg 2014;118:153–67.
20. Chia YT, Arulkumaran S, Chua S, et al. Effectiveness of transcutaneous electric nerve stimulator for pain relief in labour. Asia Oceania J Obstet Gynaecol 1990; 16:145–51.
21. Abboud TK, Gangolly J, Mosaad P, et al. Isoflurane in obstetrics. Anesth Analg 1989;68:388–91.
22. Yeo ST, Holdcroft A, Yentis SM, et al. Analgesia with sevoflurane during labour: II. Sevoflurane compared with Entonox for labour analgesia. Br J Anaesth 2007;98: 110–5.
23. Waldenström U, Irestedt L. Obstetric pain relief and its association with remembrance of labor pain at two months and one year after birth. J Psychosom Obstet Gynaecol 2006;27:147–56.
24. Ranta P, Jouppila P, Spalding M, et al. Parturients' assessment of water blocks, pethidine, nitrous oxide, paracervical and epidural blocks in labour. Int J Obstet Anesth 1994;3:193–8.

25. Holdcroft A, Morgan M. An assessment of the analgesic effect in labour of pethidine and 50 per cent nitrous oxide in oxygen (Entonox). J Obstet Gynaecol Br Commonw 1974;81:603–7.

26. Dammer U, Weiss C, Raabe E, et al. Introduction of inhaled nitrous oxide and oxygen for pain management during labour - evaluation of patients' and midwives' satisfaction. Geburtshilfe Frauenheilkd 2014;74:656–60.

27. Jones PL, Rosen M, Mushin WW, et al. Methoxyflurane and nitrous oxide as obstetric analgesics. I. A comparison by continuous administration. Br Med J 1969; 3:255–9.

28. Jones PL, Rosen M, Mushin WW, et al. Methoxyflurane and nitrous oxide as obstetric analgesics. II. A comparison by self-administered intermittent inhalation. Br Med J 1969;3:259–62.

29. Abboud TK, Shnider SM, Wright RG, et al. Enflurane analgesia in obstetrics. Anesth Analg 1981;60:133–7.

30. Abboud TK, Swart F, Zhu J, et al. Desflurane analgesia for vaginal delivery. Acta Anaesthesiol Scand 1995;39:259–61.

31. Harrison RF, Shore M, Woods T, et al. A comparative study of 1970 transcutaneous electrical nerve stimulation (TENS), entonox, pethidine + promazine and lumbar epidural for pain relief in labor. Acta Obstet Gynecol Scand 1987;66:9–14.

32. Leong EW, Sivanesaratnam V, Oh LL, et al. Epidural analgesia in primigravidae in spontaneous labour at term: a prospective study. J Obstet Gynaecol Res 2000; 26:271–5.

33. Henry A, Nand SL. Intrapartum pain management at the royal hospital for women. Aust N Z J Obstet Gynaecol 2004;44:307–13.

34. Angle P, Landy CK, Charles C, et al. Phase 1 development of an index to measure the quality of neuraxial labour analgesia: exploring the perspectives of childbearing women. Can J Anaesth 2010;57:468–78.

35. Collis RE, Davies DW, Aveling W. Randomised comparison of combined spinal-epidural and standard epidural analgesia in labour. Lancet 1995;345:1413–6.

36. Capogna G, Alahuhta S, Celleno D, et al. Maternal expectations and experiences of labour pain and analgesia: a multicentre study of nulliparous women. Int J Obstet Anesth 1996;5:229–35.

37. Hodnett ED. Pain and women's satisfaction with the experience of childbirth: a systematic review. Am J Obstet Gynecol 2002;186:S160–72.

38. Gulliver BG, Fisher J, Roberts L. A new way to assess pain in laboring women: replacing the rating scale with a "coping" algorithm. Nurs Womens Health 2008;12:404–8.

39. Roberts L, Gulliver B, Fisher J, et al. The coping with labor algorithm: an alternate pain assessment tool for the laboring woman. J Midwifery Womens Health 2010; 55:107–16.

40. Attanasio L, Kozhimannil KB, Jou J, et al. Women's experiences with neuraxial labor analgesia in the Listening to Mothers II Survey: a content analysis of open-ended responses. Anesth Analg 2015;121:974–80.

41. Alexander JM, Sharma SK, McIntire DD, et al. Intensity of labor pain and cesarean delivery. Anesth Analg 2001;92:1524–8.

42. Hess PE, Pratt SD, Soni AK, et al. An association between severe labor pain and cesarean delivery. Anesth Analg 2000;90:881–6.

43. Richardson MG, Lopez BM, Baysinger CL, et al. Nitrous oxide during labor: maternal satisfaction does not depend exclusively on analgesic effectiveness. Anesth Analg 2016, in press.

44. Minnich ME. Childbirth preparation and non-pharmacologic analgesia. In: Chestnut DH, Wong CA, Tsen LC, et al, editors. Chestnut's obstetric anesthesia: principles and practice. 5th edition. Philadelphia: Elsevier-Saunders; 2014. p. 427–37.
45. Smith CA, Levett KM, Collins CT, et al. Relaxation techniques for pain management in labour. Cochrane Database Syst Rev 2011;(12):CD009514.
46. Clett ER, Burns E. Immersion in water in labor and birth. Cochrane Database Syst Rev 2009;(2):CD0000111.
47. Smith CA, Collins CT, Crowther CA, et al. Acupuncture or acupressure for pain management in labor. Cochrane Database Syst Rev 2011;(7):CD009232.
48. Dowswell T, Bedwell C, Lavencer T, et al. Transcutaneous electrical nerve stimulation (TENS) for pain relief in labor. Cochrane Database Syst Rev 2009;(2):CD007214.
49. Derry S, Straube S, More RA, et al. Intracutaneous or subcutaneous sterile water injection compared with blinded control for pain management in labor. Cochrane Database Syst Rev 2012;(1):CD009107.
50. Ullman R, Smith LA, Burns E, et al. Parenteral opioids for maternal pain relief in labour. Cochrane Database Syst Rev 2010;(8):CD007396.
51. Olofsson C, Ekblom A, Ekman-Ordeberg G, et al. Lack of analgesic effect of systematically administered morphine or pethidine on labour pain. Br J Obstet Gynaecol 1996;103:968–72.
52. Douma MR, Verwey RA, Kam-Endtz CE, et al. Obstetric analgesia: a comparison of patient controlled meperidine, remifentanil, and fentanyl in labour. Br J Anaesth 2010;104:209–15.
53. Van de Velde M, Carvalho B. Remifentanil for labor analgesia: an evidence-based narrative review. Int J Obstet Anesth 2016;25:66–74.
54. Balki M, Kasocdekar S, Dhumne S, et al. Remifentanil patient-controlled analgesia for labour: optimizing drug delivery regimens. Can J Anaesth 2007;54: 626–33.
55. Volmanen P, Akuari E, Raudaskoski T, et al. Comparison of remifentanil and nitrous oxide in labour analgesia. Acta Anaesthesiol Scand 2005;49:453–8.
56. Blair JM, Hill DA, Fee JPH. Patient controlled analgesia for labour using remifentanil: a feasibility study. Br J Anaesth 2001;87:415–20.
57. Lucas DN, Siemaszko O, Yentis SM. Maternal hypoxaemia associated with the use of Entonox in labour. Int J Obstet Anesth 2000;9:270–2.
58. Einarsson S, Stenqvist O, Bengtsson A, et al. Gas kinetics during nitrous oxide analgesia for labour. Anaesthesia 1996;51:449–52.
59. Griffin RP, Reynolds F. Maternal hypoxaemia during labour and delivery: the influence of analgesia and effect on neonatal outcome. Anaesthesia 1995;50:151–6.
60. Paech MJ. The King Edward Memorial Hospital 1,000 mother survey of methods of pain relief in labour. Anaesth Intensive Care 1991;19:393–9.
61. Arthurs GJ, Rosen M. Self-administered intermittent nitrous oxide analgesia for labour. Enhancement of effect with continuous nasal inhalation of 50 per cent nitrous oxide (Entonox). Anaesthesia 1979;34:301–9.
62. Westling F, Milsom I, Zetterström H, et al. Effects of nitrous oxide/oxygen inhalation on the maternal circulation during vaginal delivery. Acta Anaesthesiol Scand 1992;36:175–81.
63. Committee on Nitrous Oxide and Oxygen Analgesia in Midwifery. Clinical trials of different concentrations of oxygen and nitrous oxide for obstetric analgesia. Report to the Medical Research Council of the Committee on Nitrous Oxide and Oxygen Analgesia in Midwifery. Br Med J 1970;1:709–13.

64. Stefani S, Hughes S, Shnider S, et al. Neonatal neurobehavioral effects of inhalation analgesia for vaginal delivery. Anesthesiology 1982;56:351–5.

65. King TL, Wong CA. Nitrous oxide for labor pain: is it a laughing matter? Anesth Analg 2014;118:12–4.

66. Jevtovic-Todorovic V, Hartman RE, Izumi Y, et al. Early exposure to common anesthetic agents causes widespread neurodegeneration in the developing rat brain and persistent learning deficits. J Neurosci 2003;23:876–82.

67. Flood P. Fetal anesthesia and brain development. Anesthesiology 2011;114: 479–80.

68. Munson ES. Transfer of nitrous oxide into body air cavities. Br J Anaesth 1974;46: 202–9.

69. Rösener M, Dichgans J. Severe combined degeneration of the spinal cord after nitrous oxide anaesthesia in a vegetarian. J Neurol Neurosurg Psychiatry 1996; 60:354–6.

70. The National Institute for Occupational Safety and Health (NIOSH). Controlling exposure to nitrous oxide during anesthetic administration. Atlanta (GA): DHHS (NIOSH) Publication; 1994. p. 94–100. Available at: http://www.cdc.gov/niosh/docs/94-100/. Accessed May 9, 2016.

71. Occupational and Health Administration. Nitrous oxide in workplace atmospheres (passive monitor). OSHA Method ID-166, 1985, revised May 1994. Available at: https://www.osha.gov/dts/sltc/methods/inorganic/id166/id166.html#reference_5.1. Accessed May 16, 2016.

72. European Society of Anaesthesiology. The current place of nitrous oxide in clinical practice: an expert opinion-based task force consensus statement of the European Society of Anaesthesiology. Eur J Anaesthesiol 2015;32:1–4.

73. Mills GH, Sing D, Longan J, et al. Nitrous oxide exposure on the labour floor. Int J Obstet Anesth 1996;5:16–24.

74. Munley AJ, Railton R, Gray WM, et al. Exposure of midwives to nitrous oxide in four hospitals. BMJ 1986;293:1063–4.

75. Chessor E, Verhoeven M, Hon CY, et al. Evaluation of a modified scavenging system to reduce occupational exposure to nitrous oxide in labor and delivery. J Occup Environ Hyg 2005;2:314–22.

76. Van Der Kooy J, De Graff JP, Kolder M, et al. A newly developed scavenging system for administration of nitrous oxide during labour: safe occupational use. Acta Anaesthesiol Scand 2012;56:920–5.

77. Buring JE, Hennekens CH, Mayrent SL, et al. Health experiences of operating room personnel. Anesthesiology 1985;62:325–30.

78. Mazze RI, Lecky JH. The health of operating room personnel. Anesthesiology 1985;62:226–8.

79. Rowland AS, Baird DD, Weinberg CR, et al. Reduced fertility among women employed as dental assistants exposed to high levels of nitrous oxide. N Engl J Med 1992;327:993–7.

80. Ahlborg G, Axelsson G, Lennart B. Shift work, nitrous oxide exposure and subfertility among Swedish midwives. Int J Epidemiol 1996;25:783–90.

81. Axelsson G, Ahlborg G, Lennart B. Shift work, nitrous oxide exposure, and spontaneous abortion among Swedish midwives. Occup Environ Med 1996;53:374–8.

82. Ratcliff A, Burs C, Gwinnutt CG. The contribution of medical nitrous oxide to the greenhouse effect. Health Trends 1991;23:119–20.

83. Ek M, Tjus K. Destruction of medical N_2O in Sweden. In: Guoxiang L, editor. Greenhouse gasses-capturing, utilization and reduction. Shanghai (China): InTech; 2012. p. 185–98.

84. American Society of Anesthesiologists Task Force on Sedation and Analgesia by Non-Anesthesiologists. Practice guidelines for sedation and analgesia by non-anesthesiologists. Anesthesiology 2002;96:1004–17.
85. Munro J. Understanding pharmacological pain relief. In: Royal College of Midwives, editors. Evidence based guidelines for midwifery-led care in labour. 2012. Available at: http://www.rcm.org.uk/college/polciy-practice/evidence-based-guidelines. Accessed May 8, 2016.
86. Volmanen P, Palomäki AJ. Alternatives to neuraxial analgesia for labor. Curr Opin Anaesthesiol 2011;24:235–41.
87. Collado V, Nicolas E, Faulks D, et al. Evaluation of safe and effective administration of nitrous oxide after a postgraduate training course. BMC Clin Pharmacol 2008;8:3.
88. Rooks JP. Safety and risks of nitrous oxide labor analgesia: a review. J Midwifery Womens Health 2011;56:557–65.
89. Boschert S. Nitrous oxide returns for labor pain management. Rockville (MD): OBG Management; 2016. Available at: http://www.obgmanagement.com/home/article/nitrous-oxide-returns-for-labor-pain-management/bc0fccea26eae13df876 29938d1dcc6c.html. Accessed May 11, 2016.
90. Stewart LS, Collins MR. Nitrous oxide for labor analgesia: clinical implications for nurses. Nurs Womens Health 2012;16:399–409.

Awareness and Aortocaval Obstruction in Obstetric Anesthesia

Nathaniel Hsu, MD[a],*, Robert R. Gaiser, MD[b]

KEYWORDS

- Awareness • Cesarean delivery • General anesthesia • Aortocaval compression
- Hypotension

KEY POINTS

- Awareness during general anesthesia is rare but has devastating consequences.
- According to a recent audit, cesarean delivery during general anesthesia has the highest risk of awareness.
- Anesthetic requirements necessary to consistently prevent awareness with recall in parturients may be unchanged despite the decrease in minimum alveolar concentration.
- Bispectral index (BIS) monitoring during the postdelivery phase may allow one to decrease the inhaled concentration of the volatile anesthetic while maintaining a BIS less than 60.
- Cardiac output and stroke volume were the greatest when term pregnant women were in left lateral tilt of 15°.
- The degree of aortocaval compression varies among pregnant patients, with not all patients being equally affected.
- For the patient requiring cardiopulmonary resuscitation, the position the patient should be placed for chest compressions is supine, due to the inability to provide adequate chest compressions with the patient tilted.

AWARENESS DURING GENERAL ANESTHESIA FOR CESAREAN DELIVERY
Introduction

The goals of general anesthesia include 4 conditions: analgesia, amnesia, akinesia, and areflexia. However, in the attempt to achieve these goals for optimal surgical conditions, amnesia may at times fail to occur. Awareness under general anesthesia, although rare, has devastating consequences for the patient (**Fig. 1**). These potential

[a] Department of Anesthesiology and Critical Care, Hospital of the University of Pennsylvania, 3400 Spruce Street, Philadelphia, PA 19104, USA; [b] Department of Anesthesiology, University of Kentucky, Lexington, KY 40506, USA
* Corresponding author. Department of Anesthesiology and Critical Care, Hospital of the University of Pennsylvania, 3400 Spruce Street, Dulles 7th Floor, Philadelphia, PA 19104.
E-mail address: Nathaniel.Hsu@uphs.upenn.edu

Anesthesiology Clin 35 (2017) 145–155
http://dx.doi.org/10.1016/j.anclin.2016.09.012

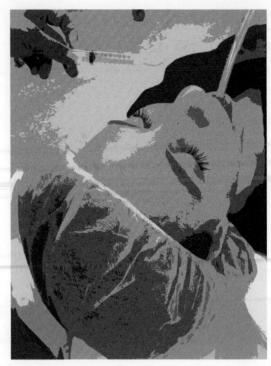

Fig. 1. Paralyzed but aware?

consequences range from fleeting memories that cause little or no psychological distress to those causing posttraumatic stress disorder. Patients may recall specific intraoperative events or conversations as well as feelings of pain, helplessness, inability to move, and panic.[1] Even though most cases of intraoperative awareness under general anesthesia do not lead to significant long-lasting sequelae, it may be extremely frightening for some individuals, subsequently resulting in a lifetime of anxiety and psychopathological effects (**Fig. 2**).

Awareness under general anesthesia can occur with or without recall of specific intraoperative events. This concept was clearly shown in a study of patients who were anesthetized with propofol and had a tourniquet placed on a forearm so that it was unaffected by neuromuscular blockade.[2] With a bispectral index (BIS) of 60 to 70 and before surgical stimulus, 66% of patients had unequivocal responses to commands. Yet, only one-quarter of those patients reported conscious recall after recovery. Therefore, it is reasonable to assume that the anesthetic state probably interferes with memory consolidation to some degree. The problem is that it is not possible to determine when or to whom awareness may affect.

There are various risk factors for awareness that have been identified: light anesthesia, history of substance abuse, history of awareness, machine malfunction, obesity, anesthetist seniority, out-of-hours operating, difficult airway management, emergencies, use of neuromuscular blockade, and type of operation (trauma, cardiac, cesarean delivery).[1,3,4] As one of the most common surgeries in the United States, cesarean delivery was performed on more than 1.2 million women in 2014.[5] Although the use of general anesthesia in obstetrics is limited (fewer than 10% of cesarean deliveries), the risk of awareness under general anesthesia is disproportionately high in

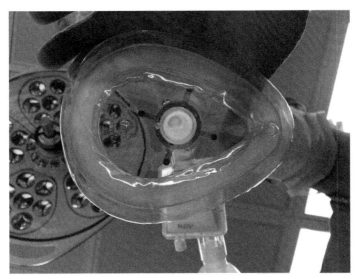

Fig. 2. Feelings of helplessness.

the obstetric population. Obstetric cases account for 0.8% of general anesthetics in the Fifth National Audit Project (NAP5) Activity Survey, but approximately 10% of reports of awareness with recall to NAP5, making it the most markedly overrepresented of all surgical specialties.[4] This disparity between the high incidence of awareness despite the low use of general anesthesia in obstetrics may be related to various patient and surgical factors.

Patient Factors That Increase the Risk of Awareness in Obstetric Anesthesia

Historically, it has been presumed that pregnant women have a hormonally mediated 25% to 40% decrease in minimum alveolar concentration (MAC), which represents the inhaled concentration of volatile anesthetic that prevents 50% of patients from moving to noxious stimuli.[6] This concept, however, is a function of the effects of anesthetics on the spinal cord rather than on the brain. Ueyama and colleagues[7] studied the effects of volatile anesthetics on the brain and discovered no differences in BIS monitoring between pregnant and nonpregnant individuals undergoing general anesthesia. They demonstrated in this electroencephalographic study that the decrease in MAC during pregnancy does not mean that volatile anesthetics have an enhanced hypnotic effect on the maternal brain. Thus, anesthetic requirements necessary to consistently prevent awareness with recall in parturients may be unchanged despite the decrease in MAC.

Labor, however, may have an effect on maternal anesthetic requirements. Laboring parturients were shown to require less sevoflurane to maintain a similar BIS value compared with their nonlaboring counterparts.[8] Additionally, Yoo and colleagues[9] demonstrated that prior labor was associated with lower intraoperative BIS values as well as reduced postoperative analgesic consumption in women undergoing cesarean delivery compared with nonlaboring women.

Other physiologic changes of pregnancy that could play a role in the higher incidence of awareness in the obstetric population include tachycardia as well as the significant increase in cardiac output at term. Tachycardia may mask the clinical signs of inadequate anesthesia, whereas the increase in cardiac output could decrease the duration of action of intravenous (IV) anesthetics, and at the same time prolong the time to establish an effective partial pressure of volatile agents.[4]

In addition, there are individual patient-specific characteristics that may lead to an increased risk for awareness among obstetric patients. These risk factors include obesity, difficult airway management, and previous history of awareness. Obesity may play a role due to its effects on drug distribution and elimination. Moreover, the incidence of maternal obesity is not only increasing but is doing so at an accelerating pace.[10]

While investigating the trends in difficult airway management, it has been noted that the incidence of failed tracheal intubations (1:224) has remained steady in obstetrics over the past 20 years despite advances in airway techniques.[11] It is not the patient's airway that places the patient at risk for awareness per se, but rather the prolonged duration of time from induction to a secured airway. Failure to administer additional anesthetics during this prolonged period may potentially lead to the patient having awareness and recall of the intubation.

Surgical Factors That Increase the Risk of Awareness in Obstetric Anesthesia

The type of surgery may play a role in determining risk of awareness in the obstetric population. Pregnant women who had cesarean deliveries under general anesthesia had a higher incidence of awareness than pregnant women under general anesthesia for other procedures; 1:670 (0.15%) versus 1:4500 (0.02%), respectively.[4]

As identified in NAP5, general anesthesia for cesarean delivery may involve many of the risk factors for awareness. These risk factors include rapid sequence induction of anesthesia, brief period between anesthetic induction and start of surgery with little time for reinforcement of the IV induction dose with a volatile agent, and a high incidence of urgent/immediate surgery often performed out-of-hours, leading to higher rates of care by less experienced providers.[4] Most cesarean deliveries under general anesthesia are nonelective and, consequently, patients' anxiety levels are likely to be high at the time of induction.[4] Additionally, due to the concern over exposure of anesthetic agents to the fetus, some institutions will prepare the abdomen with aseptic solution and drape before induction of anesthesia so as to proceed to skin incision as soon as the patient is intubated. Laryngoscopy, intubation, and skin incision were shown to be the times when parturients had the highest incidence of conscious responses to command.[12] Therefore, it should not be surprising that the NAP5 report found that all the experiences in obstetric cases concerned awareness at induction or soon thereafter.[4]

Electroencephalographic Monitoring in Obstetric Anesthesia

BIS monitoring has been used throughout the literature as a tool to determine anesthetic depth; however, processed electroencephalograph (EEG) monitors have not been sufficiently validated in pregnant patients.[13] Additionally, its reliability in emergent situations such as with rapid sequence inductions may be questionable due to its lag time of approximately 25 seconds in the speed of onset of monitoring from the awake to the general anesthetic state and vice versa.[14]

In one study comparing BIS and the isolated forearm technique (IFT), Zand and colleagues[12] noted that 49% of parturients had a conscious IFT response during one of the following events: laryngoscopy, intubation, or skin incision. They found that the BIS monitor was an unreliable and poor predictor of consciousness. In the attempt to improve the likelihood of unconsciousness in these early phases of surgery, they suggest that lower than previously recommended values (BIS <27) are needed to avoid positive IFT responses during laryngoscopy, intubation, and skin incision.

BIS monitoring may be helpful in the setting of postpartum hemorrhage as a result of uterine atony. In this particular instance, BIS monitoring during the postdelivery phase may allow one to decrease the inhaled concentration of the volatile anesthetic while maintaining a BIS less than 60. Alternatively, it could also allow one to convert to a total IV anesthetic (TIVA) regimen to minimize any anesthetic effects on uterine tone. The use of BIS monitoring in TIVA is one distinct arena in which it has been shown to be a more useful monitor of anesthetic depth.[15,16] However, its use in postpartum hemorrhage as well as TIVA may need to be validated.

Induction phase

There are perhaps a few variations in the induction of general anesthesia in cesarean deliveries that could explain the disproportionately high incidence of awareness in obstetrics. These differences include the limited amount of time to supplement the waning IV induction dose with volatile agent before skin incision, the omission of opioids at induction and sedative premedications, the frequent use yet sometimes inappropriately low doses of induction agent, and the universal use of neuromuscular blockade.[4]

Despite the unavailability of thiopental in the United States, interestingly, 93% of survey respondents in the United Kingdom stated that they continue to use thiopental for induction, yet 58% would support a change to propofol.[17] The use of low doses of thiopental (less than 4 mg/kg) were found in 50% of the obstetric awareness cases in NAP5, and the investigators suggested a dose of 5 mg/kg for the healthy parturient due to previously observed lower rates of awareness with 5 to 7 mg/kg rather than 3 to 4 mg/kg.[4,18] While studying induction doses of propofol (2.4 mg/kg) compared with thiopental (5 mg/kg), Celleno and colleagues[19] discovered a significantly greater incidence (50% vs 10%) of rapid low-voltage waves, suggestive of a light plane of anesthesia, with propofol administration. However, other studies in the nonobstetric population have suggested that propofol (2 mg/kg) tends to be associated with lower BIS values on intubation compared with thiopental (4 or 5 mg/kg).[20,21] Another group studying recovery of spontaneous ventilation after apnea also reported that when thiopental 5 mg/kg and suxamethonium 1 mg/kg were administered to volunteers and allowed to wear off, 58% experienced awareness while still paralyzed.[22] Even though some of these studies were not performed in the obstetric population, they still raise concerns over the choice of induction agent as well as optimal dosing.

The deliberate avoidance of opioids and sedatives before delivery has been due to concerns over adverse neonatal effects. Nevertheless, low-dose anxiolytics or sedatives before delivery have not shown to produce negative neonatal consequences. Senel and Mergan[23] demonstrated both maternal and neonatal safety with the use of IV midazolam 0.025 mg/kg. Frölich and colleagues[24] also found no associated adverse effects when parturients were administered fentanyl 1 μg/kg and midazolam 0.02 mg/kg IV.

Maintenance phase

The traditional use of low-concentration (0.5 MAC) of a halogenated volatile anesthetic agent delivered in 50% nitrous oxide has been driven by concerns over neonatal depression and uterine atony. Yet studies that have examined this anesthetic regimen have shown potentially inadequate anesthetic depth as evidenced by BIS values that are not consistently below 60.[25,26] One group studying anesthetic dosing found that the median effective end-tidal concentration (EC_{50}) of sevoflurane to achieve a BIS lower than 60 in 50% of parturients at the time of skin incision and delivery is 1.22%.[27]

Of course, there should be an appropriate concern for the use of higher doses of halogenated volatile anesthetics because this class of drugs has been shown to decrease uterine muscle contractility in a dose-dependent fashion.[28] This in vitro study demonstrated that volatile anesthetic concentrations of between 1.4 and 2.3 MAC are needed to achieve a 50% decrease in uterine muscle contractile amplitude and frequency. However, when more modest doses of inhaled anesthetics have been used, deleterious maternal or neonatal effects have not been noted.[25,27,29–31] Therefore, an end-tidal MAC of 0.8 for halogenated volatile anesthetics should be targeted to decrease the risk of awareness.[30] Initial high fresh-gas flows should be encouraged to increase the inspired gas concentration, and thus leading to a more rapid increase in alveolar concentration.

Looking in the Past and to the Future

In the obstetric population, the incidence of awareness was previously reported to be as high as 4% in the 1970s when obstetric procedures were performed with thiopental for induction and nitrous oxide for maintenance, but the rates of awareness have subsequently decreased tremendously with the addition of a halogenated volatile anesthetic to nitrous oxide.[32,33] One prospective trial showed an incidence of awareness of 0.26%,[34] whereas the NAP5 investigators, who did not use the Brice Protocol to interview patients for recall, had a lower incidence (0.15%) for cesarean deliveries under general anesthesia because they relied on spontaneous patient reporting.[4] Further work still needs to be done to clarify the incidence of awareness in this high-risk patient population.

Additionally, the dosage of induction agents had increased in the past with a subsequent decrease in the incidence of awareness. Perhaps higher doses of induction drugs may need to be evaluated once again. Even though more information is needed to elucidate the optimal dosing regimen for induction agents, the difficulty in determining dosing is in part due to challenges in monitoring for awareness. Depth of anesthetic monitoring with processed EEG needs further validation to identify the awareness threshold in the obstetric population.

The safe use of low-dose sedatives and opioids before neuraxial anesthesia for cesarean delivery has been shown already; however, its safety profile in patients undergoing general anesthesia should be studied as well. Timing and dosing of these medications needs to be examined further.

Although more data on intravenous anesthetic agents is a must, it is still necessary to investigate the inhaled agents as well. Areas of work include defining the EC_{95} of the volatile anesthetic agents in parturients and identifying the safe minimum inspired air fraction level so as to achieve the maximum fraction of nitrous oxide.

Last, despite most general anesthetics proceeding smoothly without incident, a single occurrence of awareness with recall may lead to a lifetime of psychological distress for that patient. If an accidental awareness event does happen, it should be promptly discussed with the patient and early supportive counseling offered to mitigate any psychological sequelae. Continued investigations, like those discussed previously, are needed to decrease the incidence of this potentially devastating anesthetic complication in this high-risk population.

AORTOCAVAL COMPRESSION
Definition and Significance

The concern with maintaining the pregnant patient in the supine position is supine hypotensive syndrome. In this situation, it is thought that the gravid uterus compresses the aorta, decreasing blood flow to the uterus. Furthermore, the gravid uterus would also compress the vena cava, reducing venous return with a resultant decrease in cardiac output.[35] This concern increases from 20 weeks' gestation until term. Furthermore, it is thought to be more severe if the patient is receiving general or neuraxial anesthesia, as both will inhibit the sympathetic nervous system and its ability to compensate. Aortocaval compression was first presented in 1943 by McLennan.[36] In this study, angiographic studies were performed in term pregnant women demonstrating the compression. Furthermore, femoral arterial and venous pressures were measured, with an increase in femoral venous pressure and a decrease in femoral arterial pressure when the patient was placed in the supine position. Given these clinical findings, the natural next step was to study whether tilting the patient to one side or the other relieved this aortocaval compression.

After the concern regarding the supine hypotensive syndrome was raised, numerous investigators studied the hemodynamic effects. In fact, some individuals raised the concern of cardiovascular collapse should a term pregnant patient assume the supine position, especially if neuraxial anesthesia was administered before assuming the supine procedure. It was estimated that 1% of 2000 patients who receive spinal anesthesia for cesarean delivery will experience cardiovascular collapse.[35] Given this concern, Wright[35] investigated 100 term pregnant patients. In this series, only 41% of the patients had a decrease in blood pressure of 10% or more when assuming the supine position. Accompanying this decrease was an increase in heart rate. More importantly, Wright[35] showed that in those patients with a decrease in blood pressure, adjusting the position to left lateral position returned the hemodynamics to baseline. A full lateral position was not necessary; rather, hemodynamics returned to baseline with a tilt as little as 20 to 30°. Although the major focus of the study was on the hypotensive syndrome, it was the first to suggest that a term pregnant patient should be placed in a lateral tilt position of 30°, especially if the patient received neuraxial anesthesia.

Tilting the Patient

The original study combined with the subsequent research in lateral tilt led to the practice of tilting the patient or using a wedge for left uterine displacement. In fact, an editorial in which the amount of left tilt was discussed, the conclusion was that it should be as much as possible.[37] The editorial focused on the adverse effects of supine positioning on the fetus, citing fetal acidosis and decreased delivery of oxygen to the fetus. The major component of the supine hypotensive syndrome was from compression of the aorta, arguing for a tilt of at least 30° to prevent this compression of the aorta. As such, it is the compression of both the aorta and the vena cava that accounted for the dangerously low blood pressure of the mother and to the compromise of the fetus.

Twenty healthy women at term had their stroke volume, arterial pressure, and cardiac output determined in various positions. In the standing position, there is no aortocaval compression with the greatest cardiac output and the highest systolic blood pressure. In the left lateral position of 45°, cardiac output was greatest with the left position as compared with the right lateral position.[38] Of note, right lateral position resulted in a greater cardiac output than the supine position (5.9 L/min vs 5.5 L/min); however, the left lateral position resulted in a greater cardiac output than the right (6.6 L/min vs 5.9 L/min). Thus, it was established that term pregnant women should not be maintained in the supine position and that they should be tilted toward the left rather than the right.

With this concept firmly established within the anesthesia community, the optimal tilt needed to be determined. Bamber and Dresner[39] studied 32 term pregnant women. Cardiac output, stroke volume, and heart rate were measured using bioimpedance cardiography. Cardiac output and stroke volume were the greatest when women were in left lateral tilt of 15°, with cardiac output being the lowest when women lay on their back (CO 7.0 L/min vs 6.5 L/min). This study established the recommended 15° left lateral tilt for pregnant women. This position also was attainable with the operating room table, as well as enabled the obstetrician to perform a cesarean delivery without major interference. Any amount greater than 15° could not be obtained with an operating room table and also was too great to allow surgery to proceed.

Using suprasternal Doppler, cardiac output was measured in 157 nonlaboring term pregnant patients who were in 0°, 7.5°, 15.0°, and full lateral tilt.[40] Cardiac output increased until 15° left lateral with no statically significant increase when going from 15° to full lateral tilt. Although cardiac output improved when going from supine to 15° left lateral tilt, the difference was not as great as described by previous investigators (6.2 L/min vs 5.9 L/min). In fact, the difference was significant because of the large number of pregnant patients studied. Given that the investigators reported the mean cardiac outputs, it becomes evident that the degree of aortocaval compression varies among pregnant patients, with not all patients being equally affected. Perhaps aortocaval compression is important in only a subset of the population. It would be important to determine which subset; however, the tilting of patients to the left 15° became established.

Does Aortocaval Compression Exist

The concept of aortocaval compression was challenged by Higuchi and colleagues.[41] These investigators used a different approach. Rather than measuring hemodynamics and guessing whether the change was from aortocaval compression, these investigators used MRI, looking at the aorta and vena cava in term pregnant women. The positions of the women were supine, 15°, 30°, and 45° tilt. The table was not tilted, rather a wedge foam was used. As expected, the vena cava was compressed with the patient in the supine position. The compression did not improve with a 15° tilt; rather it did not improve until a 30° tilt was achieved. The only means to prevent compression of the vena cava is to have the patient tilted to 30°, a position in which it is not possible to operate. Furthermore, in the supine position, the aorta was not compressed. The results of this study suggest aortocaval compression is only caval compression in the supine position. It is important to note that the patient population had an average height of 160 ± 5 cm and a weight of 57 ± 8 kg. This population weighs less than the average population in the United States. Despite this difference, the study does challenge the premise that parturients, especially when anesthetized, must be maintained in a left lateral tilt of 15°.

Obese patients

The results of Higuchi and colleagues[41] occurred in thin patients. The literature suggests that the same may not apply to the obese population. Body weight has a negative correlation with the umbilical cord pH of the neonate born to mothers during spinal anesthesia.[42] In a retrospective study of 5742 women undergoing elective cesarean delivery during spinal anesthesia, body mass index (BMI) had a negative correlation with umbilical cord pH.[43] For every 10-unit increase in BMI, the umbilical cord pH decreased by 0.01 and the base deficit increased by 0.26 mmol/L. Those pregnant patients with a BMI of 40 kg/m^2 or greater had a mean umbilical cord pH of 7.220. In this group, 7.7% of the morbidly obese patients had an umbilical cord pH less than 7.10. Although some postulate it may be the longer incision to delivery time, it also may be due to aortocaval compression, which may be exaggerated in the obese pregnant patients. Examining anesthetic outcomes in 142 morbidly obese pregnant patients receiving spinal anesthesia revealed a greater incidence of profound hypotension in the morbidly obese pregnant patients.[43]

Cardiopulmonary resuscitation

The guidelines for cardiopulmonary resuscitation for the pregnant patient have recently been updated. When initiating cardiopulmonary resuscitation in the pregnant patient, chest compressions should be performed at a rate of 100/min at a depth of 2 inches and a compression-ventilation ratio of 30:2. Interestingly, the patient should be placed in the supine position for chest compressions, due to the inability to provide adequate chest compressions with the patient tilted.[44] Left uterine displacement is still recommended but it should be performed manually.

SUMMARY

It is standard to tilt pregnant patients receiving anesthesia to the left to prevent aortocaval compression. It appears that not all patients will experience aortocaval compression when in the supine position and that tilting the patient to the left will relieve compression of the vena cava. Obesity most likely increases the risk of aortocaval compression. Unfortunately, due to the body habitus, it is not possible to achieve adequate tilt to reduce the compression. When cardiopulmonary resuscitation is performed, the pregnant patient is placed SUPINE, with left uterine displacement maintained manually. Despite not all patients experiencing aortocaval compression when supine, all patients receiving anesthesia will be placed in left tilt. With the increasing use of transthoracic echocardiography, it will become possible to identify the patient who experiences aortocaval compression and to adjust the tilt to minimize the effects from the compression.

REFERENCES

1. Ghoneim MM, Block RI, Haffarnan M, et al. Awareness during anesthesia: risk factors, causes and sequelae: a review of reported cases in the literature. Anesth Analg 2009;108:527–35.
2. Kerssens C, Klein J, Bonke B. Awareness: monitoring versus remembering what happened. Anesthesiology 2003;99:570.
3. Bischoff P, Rundshagen I. Awareness under general anesthesia. Dtsch Arztebl 2011;108:1–7.
4. Pandit JJ, Cook TM. Accidental Awareness during General Anaesthesia in the United Kingdom and Ireland. 5th National Audit Project of the Royal College of Anaesthetists and the Association of Anaesthetists of Great Britain and Ireland. 2014. Available at: http://www.nationalauditprojects.org.uk/NAP5report. Accessed May 31, 2016.
5. Births – method of delivery. CDC. 2015. Available at: http://www.cdc.gov/nchs/fastats/delivery.htm. Accessed May 27, 2016.
6. Palahniuk RJ, Shnider SM, Eger EI 2nd. Pregnancy decreases the requirement for inhaled anesthetic agents. Anesthesiology 1974;41:82–3.
7. Ueyama H, Hagihara S, Takashina M, et al. Pregnancy does not enhance volatile anesthetic sensitivity on the brain: an electroencephalographic analysis. Anesthesiology 2010;113:577–84.

8. Erden V, Erkalp K, Yangin Z, et al. The effect of labor on sevoflurane requirements during cesarean delivery. Int J Obstet Anesth 2011;20:17–21.
9. Yoo KY, Jeong CW, Kang MW, et al. Bispectral index values during sevoflurane-nitrous oxide general anesthesia in women undergoing cesarean delivery: a comparison between women with and without prior labor. Anesth Analg 2008;106:1827–32.
10. Helsehurst N, Ells LJ, Simpson H, et al. Trends in maternity obesity incidence, rates, demographic predictors, and health inequalities in 38,821 women over a 15-year period. BJOG 2007;114:187–94.
11. Quinn AC, Milne D, Columb M, et al. Failed tracheal intubation in obstetric anaesthesia: 2 yr national case-control study in the UK. Br J Anaesth 2013;110:74–80.
12. Zand F, Hadavi SMR, Chohedri A, et al. Survey on the adequacy of depth of anaesthesia with bispectral index and isolated forearm technique in elective caesarean section under general anaesthesia with sevoflurane. Br J Anaesth 2014;112:871–8.
13. Sanders RD, Avidan MS. Evidence is lacking for interventions proposed to prevent unintended awareness during general anesthesia for cesarean delivery. Anesth Analg 2010;110:972–3.
14. Zanner R, Pilge S, Kochs EF, et al. Time delay of electroencephalogram index calculation: analysis of cerebral state, bispectral, and Narcotrend indices using perioperatively recorded electroencephalographic signals. Br J Anaesth 2009; 103:394–9.
15. Zhang C, Xu L, Ma YQ, et al. Bispectral index monitoring prevent awareness during total intravenous anesthesia: a prospective, randomized, double-blinded, multi-center controlled trial. Chin Med J (Engl) 2011;124:3664–9.
16. Myles PS, Leslie K, McNeil J, et al. Bispectral index monitoring to prevent awareness during anaesthesia: the B-Aware randomised controlled trial. Lancet 2004; 363:1757–63.
17. Murdoch H, Scrutton M, Laxton CH. Choice of anaesthetic agents for caesarean section: a UK survey of current practice. Int J Obstet Anesth 2013;22:31–5.
18. Lyons G, Macdonald R. Awareness during caesarean section. Anaesthesia 1991; 46:62–4.
19. Celleno D, Capogna G, Emanuelli M, et al. Which induction drug for cesarean section? A comparison of thiopental sodium, propofol, and midazolam. J Clin Anesth 1993;5:284–8.
20. Sie MY, Goh PK, Chan L, et al. Bispectral index during modified rapid sequence induction using thiopentone or propofol and rocuronium. Anaesth Intensive Care 2004;32:28–30.
21. Beck CE, Pohl B, Janda M, et al. Depth of anaesthesia during intubation: comparison between propofol and thiopentone. Anaesthesist 2006;55:401–6.
22. Heier T, Feiner JR, Lin J, et al. Hemoglobin desaturation after succinylcholine-induced apnea: a study of the recovery of spontaneous ventilation in healthy volunteers. Anesthesiology 2001;94:754–9.
23. Senel AC, Mergan F. Premedication with midazolam prior to caesarean section has no neonatal adverse effects. Braz J Anesthesiol 2014;64:16–21.
24. Frölich MA, Burchfield DJ, Euliano TY, et al. A single dose of fentanyl and midazolam prior to cesarean section have no adverse neonatal effects. Can J Anaesth 2006;53:79–85.
25. Chin KJ, Yeo SW. Bispectral index values at sevoflurane concentrations of 1% and 1.5% in lower segment cesarean delivery. Anesth Analg 2004;98:1140–4.
26. Yeo SN, Lo WK. Bispectral index in assessment of adequacy of general anaesthesia for lower segment caesarean section. Anaesth Intensive Care 2002;30:36–40.

27. Chin KJ, Yeo SW. A BIS-guided study of sevoflurane requirements for adequate depth of anaesthesia in caesarean section. Anaesthesia 2004;59:1064–8.

28. Yoo KY, Lee JC, Yoon MH, et al. The effects of volatile anesthetics on spontaneous contractility of isolated human pregnant uterine muscle: a comparison among sevoflurane, desflurane, isoflurane, and halothane. Anesth Analg 2006; 103:443–7.

29. Ittichaikulthol W, Sriswasdi S, Prachanpanich N, et al. Bispectral index in assessment of 3% and 4.5% desflurane in 50% N2O for caesarean section. J Med Assoc Thai 2007;90:1546–50.

30. Yildiz K, Dogru K, Dalgic H, et al. Inhibitory effects of desflurane and sevoflurane on oxytocin-induced contractions of isolated pregnant human myometrium. Acta Anaesthesiol Scand 2005;49:1355–9.

31. Robins K, Lyons G. Intraoperative awareness during general anesthesia for cesarean delivery. Anesth Analg 2009;109:886–90.

32. Moir DD. Anaesthesia for caesarean section: an evaluation of a method using low concentrations of halothane and 50 percent of oxygen. Br J Anaesth 1970;42: 136–42.

33. Crawford JS. Awareness during operative obstetrics under general anaesthesia. Br J Anaesth 1971;43:179–82.

34. Paech MJ, Scott KL, Clavisi O, et al, The ANZCA Trials group. A prospective study of awareness and recall associated with general anaesthesia for caesarean section. Int J Obstet Anesth 2008;17:298–303.

35. Wright L. Postural hypotension in late pregnancy: "The supine hypotensive syndrome". BMJ 1962;1:760–2.

36. McLennan CE. Antecubital and femoral venous pressure in normal and toxemic pregnancy. Am J Obstet Gynecol 1943;45:568–91.

37. Kinsella SM, Whitwam JG, Spencer JAD. Reducing aortocaval compression: how much tilt is enough? Do as much as possible in the lateral position. BMJ 1992; 305:539–40.

38. Armstrong S, Fernando R, Columb M, et al. Cardiac index in term pregnant women in the sitting, lateral, and supine positions: an observational, crossover study. Anesth Analg 2011;113:318–22.

39. Bamber JH, Dresner M. Aortocaval compression in pregnancy: the effect of changing the degree and direction of lateral tilt on maternal cardiac output. Anesth Analg 2003;97:256–8.

40. Lee SWY, Khaw KS, Kee WDN, et al. Haemodynamic effects from aortocaval compression at different angles of lateral tilt in non-labouring term pregnant women. Br J Anaesth 2012;109:950–6.

41. Higuchi H, Takagi S, Zhang K, et al. Effect of lateral tilt angle on the volume of the abdominal aorta and inferior vena cava in pregnant and nonpregnant women determined by magnetic resonance imaging. Anesthesiology 2015;122:286–93.

42. Edwards RK, Cantu J, Cliver S, et al. The association of maternal obesity with fetal pH and base deficit at cesarean delivery. Obstet Gynecol 2013;122:262–7.

43. Vricella LK, Louis JM, Mercer BM, et al. Anesthesia complications during scheduled cesarean delivery for morbidly obese women. Am J Obstet Gynecol 2010; 203:276.e1-5.

44. Lavonas EJ, Drennan IR, Gabrielli A, et al. Special circumstances of resuscitation: 2015 American Heart Association guidelines update for cardiopulmonary resuscitation and emergency cardiovascular care. Circulation 2015;132:S501–18.

Postdural Puncture Headache

An Evidence-Based Approach

Robert R. Gaiser, MD

KEYWORDS

- Accidental dural puncture • Postdural puncture headache • Epidural blood patch
- Intrathecal catheter

KEY POINTS

- According to the International Headache Society, a postdural puncture headache (PDPHA) is any headache that develops within 5 days of dural puncture and is not better accounted for by any other cause. It is usually accompanied by neck stiffness and subjective hearing symptoms.
- Headache and backache may persist after accidental dural puncture beyond 6 weeks in a small subset of the population.
- Obesity may decrease the incidence of headache after accidental dural puncture. It definitely does not increase the risk of a patient developing a headache after accidental dural puncture.
- The incidence of PDPHA is greater in women who deliver vaginally compared with those who deliver by cesarean delivery.
- The data concerning prophylactic epidural blood patch are conflicting. If an epidural catheter is resited after accidental dural puncture and the placement was difficult, a prophylactic epidural blood patch may be helpful.

INTRODUCTION

Headache is the most common complication after neuraxial anesthesia, especially in obstetric anesthesia. The problem with headaches in postpartum parturients is that the headache may be due to one of several causes, as outlined in **Box 1**.[1] Most non-anesthesiologists automatically assume that a headache in a parturient who received neuraxial anesthesia is due to the anesthetic. The majority of headaches occurring in the postpartum period, however, are due to tension, with preeclampsia being the second leading reason. PDPHA is a leading cause of lawsuits.[2] It is surprising that a condition that may reasonably be managed results in lawsuits. This fact reflects the disappointment patients experience when this complication occurs as well as that

Department of Anesthesiology, University of Kentucky, Lexington, KY 40506, USA
E-mail address: robert.gaiser@uky.edu

Anesthesiology Clin 35 (2017) 157–167
http://dx.doi.org/10.1016/j.anclin.2016.09.013   **anesthesiology.theclinics.com**

Box 1
Causes of postpartum headaches
Stress
Preeclamspsia
Dural puncture
Caffeine withdrawal
Pain
Breastfeeding

they feel that they have not received appropriate follow-up. Given this background, it is not surprising that there has been significant investigation into the diagnosis and management of PDPHA.

PATHOPHYSIOLOGY OF POSTDURAL PUNCTURE HEADACHE

A PDPHA is due to loss of cerebrospinal fluid. In patients with accidental dural puncture who had MRI, headache was associated with more extensive and more rostral distributions of periradicular leaks and epidural collections.[3] Furthermore, these leaks were not restricted to the level of the dural defect, although the majority did remain within the location of the accidental dural puncture. According to the International Headache Society, a PDPHA is any headache that develops within 5 days of dural puncture and is not better accounted for by any other cause. It is usually accompanied by neck stiffness and subjective hearing symptoms.[4] It also usually remits spontaneously within 2 weeks or after sealing of the leak with an epidural blood patch. These diagnostic criteria are different from the criteria established in 2012 in which the criteria included worsening within 15 minutes of assuming the upright position and disappearing within 15 minutes of assuming the supine position. The headache typically occurs in the frontal and occipital areas and also has a positional component. Although it generally occurs within 48 hours of the dural puncture, it may occur later than 3 days after the dural puncture in 25% of the cases. Although an overwhelming majority of cases develop a positional headache where assuming the upright position worsens the headache, there are a minority of patients who develop an atypical headache in which the headache is worse with assuming the recumbent position. In a series of 27,064 neuraxial anesthetics in pregnant patients, 142 patients experienced an accidental dural puncture; 8 of these patients developed this atypical headache.[5] The headache did have visual disturbances accompanying it; however, it worsened with assuming a recumbent position and improved with assuming the upright position. Furthermore, the headache improved with an epidural blood patch. All these factors, except the positional aspects, suggested the headache was due to the dural puncture. The importance of this study is to remember that not all headaches from dural puncture exhibit the typical change in symptoms with assuming various positions.

Other symptoms that accompany a PDPHA include nausea, vomiting, neck stiffness, visual disturbances, and hearing alteration. Visual disturbances (blurred vision or double vision) are due to dysfunction of the extraocular muscles from transient paralysis of the cranial nerves of the eye (III, IV, and VI). These symptoms occur due to traction on the nerve from the downward displacement of the cranial contents. Of these nerves, cranial nerve VI is the most frequently affected because of its acute angulation within the cranium with the acute angulation near a point of fixation, placing the nerve at the greatest risk of traction injury.[6] The anatomic course of this nerve with its 90° bend over the petrous bone makes it susceptible to injury from traction. Symptoms consist of blurred or double vision, sensitivity to light, and trouble focusing. On physical examination, the patient has impaired ocular abduction with the eye adducting when the patient looks straight ahead. Cranial nerve VIII is also affected. The inner ear connects to the subarachnoid space through the cochlear aqueduct. If there is a loss of cerebrospinal fluid from the subarachnoid space, cerebrospinal fluid goes from the perilymph of the inner ear to the subarachnoid space through the cochlear aqueduct. This endolymphatic hydrops disrupts the hair cells within the inner ear, resulting in a hearing alteration. The individual typically experiences hearing alteration within low frequencies with no effect from sounds of the high frequencies.[7] This alteration in hearing may persist for a long period after accidental dural puncture; 60 women with accidental dural puncture treated with epidural blood patch had auditory function assessed 2 to 5 years later. There was a small minor hearing loss in pure tone audiometry years after the accidental dural puncture and epidural blood patch.[8] This small hearing loss had minor clinical significance.

Incidence

The incidence of headache after dural puncture was established by the Serious Complication Repository (SCORE) project of the Society for Obstetric Anesthesia and Perinatology.[9] In this study, 30 institutions participated, with each institution reporting the number of anesthetics and complications. As such, it was possible to determine an incidence of complications in obstetric anesthesia. The total number of postdural puncture headaches was 1647 of the 237,437 neuraxial anesthetics. The denominator included both spinal anesthetics and accidental dural punctures accompanying epidural anesthesia. Using these numbers, the incidence of PDPHA is 1:144 neuraxial anesthetics. Because this number included spinal anesthesia, it is not possible to determine the incidence of headache accompanying accidental dural puncture. A better indication of the risk is to analyze those requiring an epidural blood patch. Of the 1647 patients with a headache, 917 required an epidural blood patch (55.7% of postdural puncture headaches). Of the patients requiring epidural blood patch, 98 of the patients required a repeat epidural blood patch (10.7%). These numbers allow concluding that if a patient develops a headache after epidural anesthesia, she is likely to require an epidural blood patch. If she receives an epidural blood patch, she has a 10% chance of requiring a repeat epidural blood patch because of a return of symptoms.

Originally, it was thought that the headache accompanying an accidental dural puncture was benign, eventually resolving on its own without treatment. There are 2 studies, however, which suggest that there may be significant long-term effects from accidental dural puncture. Webb and colleagues[10] examined 40 individuals who had an accidental dural puncture with a 17-gauge Tuohy needle. Assessments included a telephone call at 12 and 24 months after delivery to determine persistence of symptomology. Of those who had an accidental dural puncture, 28% of this group reported a chronic headache (compared with 5% in the control group). Within the accidental dural puncture group, 5 of the 25 patients who received an epidural blood patch had a headache 1 year later compared with 6 of the 15 patients who did not receive an epidural blood patch. As such, accidental dural puncture with a large-bore needle has significant consequences beyond the initial headache period; although an epidural blood patch reduces the chance of developing a chronic headache, it does not completely prevent it. These results were confirmed by a subsequent study. Parturients with an accidental dural puncture with 17-gauge Tuohy needle were followed for 6 weeks after the incident.[11] In this group of 308 parturients, 87% had a headache whereas 47.2% had backache. The investigators also determined whether these symptoms were present prior to the accidental dural puncture. Only 16.7% of patients had a headache whereas 16.7% had a backache. This increase in the incidence of symptoms at 6 weeks suggests that accidental dural puncture does have consequences beyond the initial 2-week period. Both of these studies serve to reinforce that headache and backache may persist after accidental dural puncture.

RISK FACTORS FOR DEVELOPMENT OF POSTDURAL PUNCTURE HEADACHE

There are various factors that affect whether a patient will develop a headache after dural puncture. There are numerous studies that have demonstrated that young age and female gender increase the risk. As such, parturients are the greatest risk population because they fulfill these risk criteria. Recently, there has been much debate as to whether obesity affects the probability of developing a headache after dural puncture. Some investigators believe that obesity decreases the risk of developing headache. In a study of 99 patients who had accidental dural puncture, those patients with a body mass index (BMI) greater than 30 kg/m^2 had a 25% incidence of headache compared with those with a BMI less than 30 kg/m^2, in which the percentage of patients with a headache was 45%.[12] Another study examined 13,2013 parturients who received neuraxial anesthesia. Of these patients, 518 had an unintentional dural puncture. If the BMI was less than 31.5 kg/m^2, the incidence of headache was 56% whereas it was 39% if the BMI was greater than 31.5 kg/m^2.[13] These results further reinforced the concept that those parturients with an increased BMI have a lower incidence of developing a headache. The need for epidural blood patch did not differ between the groups, suggesting that there was no difference in the incidence of severe headache between the 2 groups. This second postulate may be more correct. In a retrospective analysis of 18,315 epidural anesthetics, 125 of the patients had an accidental dural puncture.[14] Of these patients, there was no difference in the incidence of headache if the BMI was greater or less than 30 kg/m^2. Although this study did not demonstrate a protective effect of obesity, all of the studies agree that obesity does not increase the risk of the patient developing a headache after accidental dural puncture.

Although obesity may or may not be protective, cesarean delivery compared with vaginal delivery is protective. This fact was discovered when the incidence of accidental dural puncture in the obstetric population was studied. The incidence of PDPHA after accidental dural puncture with a Tuohy needle was 60%, much less than expected. It is not surprising, however, when considering that an anesthesia provider takes care of 2 types of patients in the labor suite: those who deliver vaginally and those who deliver by cesarean delivery. The risk of developing a headache after accidental dural puncture is different in these populations. In 1 study of 33 patients with accidental dural puncture, 23 of them pushed during the second stage of labor whereas the other 10 patients delivered via cesarean delivery prior to the second stage.[15] One patient in the cesarean delivery group developed a PDPHA and did not require an epidural blood patch, whereas 16 patients in the vaginal delivery group developed a headache, with 13 of the 16 patients requiring an epidural blood patch. There was a moderate correlation between the length of time spent pushing and the development of a headache. In another study of 64 patients with accidental dural puncture, 51 of the patients delivered vaginally whereas 13 of the patients had a cesarean delivery.[16] The percentage of patients without a headache was higher in the cesarean delivery group (80% vs 15%). Finally, another study investigated the effect of neuraxial technique after inadvertent dural puncture.[17] In this study of 235 women who experienced inadvertent dural puncture during attempted epidural anesthesia, cesarean delivery decreased the incidence of PDPHA by 35%. These studies suggest that bearing down during the second stage may increase cerebrospinal fluid loss or increase the size of the dural rent. Either way, it is clear that accidental dural puncture in a patient who receives cesarean delivery is much less than those patients deliver vaginally. Practitioners do not alter the management of labor of patients with accidental dural puncture but realize that these patients are at a higher risk of developing a headache if a vaginal delivery occurs.

In regard to epidural catheter placement, there has been much debate concerning the choice of loss of resistance technique. Many practitioners prefer air whereas others prefer saline. It seems that the use of air may also increase the probability of the patient developing a headache if accidental dural puncture occurs. In a study of 2975 patients who received a total of 3730 epidural injections, 1812 had the space identified by loss of resistance to air whereas the rest had loss of resistance to saline.[18] There was no difference in the incidence of accidental dural puncture (2.2% in both groups). The incidence of headache, however, was markedly different, 34% versus 10%. This difference only persisted for the first 24 hours after accidental dural puncture and was not different after 24 hours. The difference may be explained by intrathecal air. This explanation also accounts for the type of headache that occurs in the first 24 hours after accidental dural puncture in which air is used in that it is sharp, diffuse, and nonpositional. To limit the headache with the loss of resistance to air as well to limit partial blockade, the smallest amount of air to identify the space should be used. Another study examined air versus saline for loss of resistance. The anesthesiologist used either air or saline based on personal preference in 929 parturients.[19] Choosing either medium for loss of resistance resulted in no difference in accidental dural puncture or in complications. This study reaffirms that either air or saline may be used safely provided that if air is used, the amount used should be the least amount possible.

PREVENTION OF POSTDURAL PUNCTURE HEADACHE

There have been several studies examining means to prevent postdural puncture headache. Currently, there is no universally accepted means to prevent headache. The methods that have been examined recently are prophylactic epidural blood patch and intrathecal catheter placement. Given the effectiveness of an epidural blood patch, it was postulated that a prophylactic epidural blood patch would prevent a headache. A prophylactic epidural blood patch involves the injection of autologous blood through the epidural catheter (usually a volume of 20 mL) prior to removing the catheter. A randomized study of 64 patients who experienced accidental dural puncture was performed.[16] Half of the patients were randomized to receive a prophylactic epidural blood patch whereas the other half received no prophylactic epidural blood patch. There was no difference in the incidence of postdural puncture headache, severity of headache, or need for subsequent epidural blood patch. The use of prophylactic epidural blood patch has been reinvestigated, however, with a different conclusion occurring. A total of 116 parturients with accidental dural puncture were randomized to either prophylactic epidural blood patch (60) or to a therapeutic epidural blood patch if needed.[20] Those patients in the prophylactic group received 15 mL to 20 mL autologous blood through the epidural catheter at least 5 hours after the last dose of epidural local anesthetic. The incidence of headache in the prophylactic epidural blood patch group was 18.3% whereas it was 79.6% in the traditional management group. Six patients in the prophylactic group required a second epidural blood patch whereas 36 patients in the conservative group required an epidural blood patch. Hence, there are 2 well-conducted studies that achieved different conclusions. There is risk to a prophylactic epidural blood patch in that all patients are exposed to epidural blood, even those who would not develop a headache. Furthermore, there is the concern of infection, although this occurrence has not been documented. Given the results from the 2 studies as well as the concerns, it is reasonable to consider a prophylactic epidural blood patch in a patient who has a difficult placement of the catheter. It may be beneficial to try a prophylactic epidural blood patch rather than subject the patient to a second attempt at epidural placement if she should develop a headache. In patients in whom epidural placement was not difficult, it may be better to wait and treat the headache rather than subject this patient to the risks of a prophylactic epidural blood patch.

The use of epidural morphine after accidental dural puncture has been proven to prevent the development of a headache.[21] A randomized double-blind trial compared the use of epidural morphine (3 mg), 2 doses 24 hours apart. The incidence of headache was significantly different, 48% in the morphine group and 25% in the control group. The incidence of side effects, such as nausea, vomiting, and pruritus, was also higher in the morphine group. The guidelines for the detection of respiratory depression after neuraxial opioids recommends that monitoring be performed for a minimum of 24 hours after administration. As such, to use epidural morphine for the prevention of headache requires that a patient remain in the hospital for 46 hours after delivery.

Given the mechanism for the development of headache after accidental dural puncture is the hole in the dura with subsequent loss of cerebrospinal fluid, it has been postulated that placement of an intrathecal catheter through the hole will limit cerebrospinal fluid loss. Ayad and colleagues[22] recommended that an epidural catheter be threaded intrathecally and left in place for 24 hours, postulating that the catheter would stimulate a fibrotic response that would result in a smaller hole. The investigators achieved an amazing success, decreasing the incidence of headache from 91.9% to 6.2% with this approach. This study affected obstetric anesthesia practice, with many practitioners now placing intrathecal catheters. In a survey to anesthesiologists in North America, 25% of respondents stated that they would place an intrathecal catheter after accidental dural puncture, with this practice not varying in other locations throughout the world, as indicated by survey responses in the United Kingdom (28% place an intrathecal catheter), in Turkey (36% place an intrathecal catheter), and in Australia (35% place an intrathecal catheter).[23–26] Despite the increase in intrathecal catheter placement, most did not achieve the results expected of an intrathecal catheter. Russell[27] randomized 115 women after accidental dural puncture either to intrathecal catheter insertion and leaving it in place for at least 24 hours after delivery to resiting the epidural catheter at another location. The insertion of an intrathecal catheter did not reduce the incidence of headache or the need for epidural blood patch. Another study used a different approach. The anesthetic records of 29,7949 patients were reviewed. There were 128 accidental dural punctures.[28] Of these patients, 39 women had an epidural catheter placed at a different level and 89 had an intrathecal catheter for at least 24 hours. Intrathecal catheter placement reduced the incidence of headache to 42% compared with 62% in the catheter resite. Both of these studies suffer from the same problem of poor criteria for the diagnosis of PDPHA and for need for epidural blood patch. To truly advance the knowledge in this area, strict criteria for a headache related to the accidental dural puncture as well as for the need for a blood patch need to be outlined and followed by all investigators. Although an intrathecal catheter may not prevent a headache, it does prevent patients from experiencing a second accidental dural puncture. In the study by Russell, more than one-third of the women in the repeat epidural catheter group suffered complications, such as a second accidental dural puncture. This occurrence suggests that in patients with difficulty in identifying the epidural space who experience an accidental dural puncture, the placement of an intrathecal catheter allows the patient to receive analgesia faster and does not place the patient at risk of a repeat accidental dural puncture. It may be prudent to place an intrathecal catheter in some patients despite the higher infectious risk. An intrathecal catheter does not affect the course of labor.[17] Although many investigators believe an intrathecal catheter definitely will function appropriately, this finding has not been consistently observed. In an observational study of intrathecal catheters versus resisting the epidural catheter, there was a higher failure rate in the intrathecal catheter group (14%) requiring catheter replacement.

TREATMENT OF POSTDURAL PUNCTURE HEADACHE

Many practitioners recommend the use of intravenous caffeine for the treatment of a headache after dural puncture, citing its cerebral vasoconstrictive properties. Despite 1 study that showed a benefit to intravenous caffeine, no subsequent study has been able to demonstrate a benefit. As such, caffeine has been shown not an effective treatment of headaches after dural puncture.[29] Another treatment recently recommended is sphenopalatine ganglion block. The sphenopalatine ganglion is an extracranial neural structure located in the pterygopalatine fossa that has both sympathetic and parasympathetic components.[30,31] It can be accessed through either a transcutaneous or a transnasal approach. The emergency medicine literature suggests that sphenopalatine ganglion block should be the first-line treatment of headache after dural puncture because it is less invasive with reasonable success. A sphenopalatine ganglion block is performed by placing a cotton-tipped swab that is soaked with lidocaine into the nostril. In 1 case series of 32 patients, 69% of the women did not require epidural blood patch. To date, there are only case series reporting the use of sphenopalatine block.

The only treatment that has been shown effective for the treatment of a headache after dural puncture is epidural blood patch. Epidural blood patch involves locating the epidural space and then injecting autologous blood, 15 mL to 20 mL. The postulated mechanism for its effectiveness is that it initially increases the pressure in the lumbar spine, compressing the thecal space and translocating cerebrospinal fluid from the spine to the cranium. Maintenance of the therapeutic effect is attributed to the clot preventing further cerebrospinal fluid loss. The use of an epidural blood patch for the treatment of headache after dural puncture is attributed to Gormley,[32] who noted that patients with a bloody lumbar puncture had a lower likelihood of developing a headache compared with those who did not. Gormley then studied 7 patients with a headache after dural puncture, with 1 of the patients being himself. All had a headache that resolved with the epidural injection of 2 mL to 3 mL of blood.

The amount of blood for an epidural blood patch has been studied. There have been numerous case series, with the amount of blood injected epidurally ranging from 6 mL to 50 mL.[33] In a randomized study, 120 parturients with accidental dural puncture with an epidural needle and with a headache were randomized to receive an epidural blood patch. The volume for the blood patch was either 15 mL, 20 mL, or 30 mL.[34] The incidence of partial relief was 51%, 41%, and 41% respectively, and of complete relief was 10%, 32%, and 26%, respectively. If a patient complained of severe back pain during injection, the final volume of blood used was limited. As such, only 81% of the parturients in the 20-mL group received the full 20 mL whereas only 54% of the parturients in the 30-mL group did. The major point of the study is that 20 mL of blood is the optimal volume for an epidural blood patch, assuming that the patient did not develop back pain or leg pain during the injection. There was no advantage to increasing the volume, with the larger amounts being limited due to back pain.

Epidural blood patch improves the visual disturbances accompanying cranial nerve IV involvement. It also improves the hearing alteration from cranial nerve VIII involvement. There is still some residual hearing alteration, which is clinically not significant or noticed by the patient. The chance of a patient developing a chronic headache is decreased. From the SCORE project, approximately 10% of epidural blood patches need to be repeated due to a return of symptoms. Complications of epidural blood patch include back pain with an estimated incidence of 80% of patients developing back pain. Another common complication is radicular pain, which is a result of the inflammatory response in the epidural space by the blood clots as well as compression of the nerve roots.[35] Other complications that have been reported include chronic adhesive arachnoiditis. Chronic adhesive arachnoiditis is an extremely rare condition consisting of back pain, leg pain, neurologic abnormalities, and MRI changes. Spinal subdural hematoma has also been described, requiring urgent neurosurgical correction.[36,37] The concern with epidural blood patch is whether it will interfere with the success of sequent epidural catheters. In a retrospective study, 29 patients with PDPHA and epidural blood patch were matched to 55 patients with dural puncture and no epidural blood patch. There was no difference in the success of subsequent epidural anesthetics between the 2 groups.[38] A patient had a failed epidural after an epidural blood patch for an accidental dural puncture. On the epidurogram in this patient, there was scarring, with contrast material restricted to T12 to L2.[39]

The management of headache after accidental dural puncture varies. This varied management extends to the literature with different definitions of PDPHA and indications for epidural blood patch. More concerning from a survey sent to members of the Society for Obstetric Anesthesia and Perinatology was the lack of follow-up of patients after accidental dural puncture. Given the conflicting data and opinions, a written protocol is important and is to be followed by all members of the department. The key components to a successful protocol after accidental dural puncture are presented in **Box 2**.

Box 2
Important components to the management of accidental dural puncture

See all patients after delivery and every day while in hospital.

Provide patients with a number to call should they develop a headache after going home.

Track all patients with symptoms consistent with postdural puncture headache.

If a patient is unable to attend to activities of daily living, offer epidural blood patch.

Consider intrathecal catheter if placement is difficult.

For epidural catheter resiting after accidental dural puncture, consider prophylactic epidural blood patch.

When doing an epidural blood patch, do not use a volume greater than 20 mL.

SUMMARY

PDPHA continues to be a problem for the obstetric anesthesia provider. There is no effective means for the prevention of a PPDH. Although some studies suggest an intrathecal catheter may be beneficial, not all studies have supported this conclusion. Given the unclear benefit, intrathecal catheters should be reserved for patients in whom repeat accidental dural puncture is not desired. Although intrathecal catheters provide rapid onset of analgesia, they do have a high failure rate necessitating replacement. Treatment of a headache after dural puncture is most effective with an epidural blood patch. For the blood patch to be effective, patients must be seen after accidental dural puncture, with practitioners following protocol.

REFERENCES

1. Stella CL, Jodicks CD, How HY, et al. Postpartum headache: is your work-up complete? Am J Obstet Gynecol 2007;196:318.e1-7.
2. Davies JM, Posner KL, Lee LA, et al. Liability associated with obstetric anesthesia: a closed claims analysis. Anesthesiology 2009;110:131–9.
3. Wang YF, Fuh JL, Lirng JF, et al. Cerebrospinal fluid leakage and headache after lumbar puncture: a prospective non-invasive imaging study. Brain 2015;138:1492–8.
4. Headache Classification Committee of the International Headache Society (IHS). The International Classification of Headache Disorders, 3rd edition (beta version). Cephalalgia 2013;33:629–808.
5. Loures V, Savoldelli G, Kern K, et al. Atypical headache following dural puncture in obstetrics. Int J Obstet Anesth 2014;23:246–52.
6. Hofer JE, Scavone BM. Cranial nerve VI palsy after dural-arachnoid puncture. Anesth Analg 2015;120:644–6.
7. Pogodzinski MS, Shallop JK, Sprung J, et al. Hearing loss and cerebrospinal fluid pressure: case report and review of the literature. Ear Nose Throat J 2009;87:144–7.
8. Darvish B, Dahlgren G, Irestedt L, et al. Auditory function following post-dural puncture headache treated with epidural blood patch. A long-term follow-up. Acta Anaesthesiol Scand 2015;59:1340–54.
9. D'Angelo R, Smiley RM, Riley ET, et al. Serious complications related to obstetric anesthesia. The serious complication repository project of the society for obstetric anesthesia and perinatology. Anesthesiology 2014;120:1505–12.
10. Webb CA, Weyker PD, Zhang L, et al. Unintentional dural puncture with a Tuohy needle increases risk of chronic headache. Anesth Analg 2012;115:124–32.
11. Ranganathan P, Golfeiz C, Phelps AL, et al. Chronic headache and backache are long-term sequelae of unintentional dural puncture in the obstetric population. J Clin Anesth 2015;27:201–6.
12. Faure E, Moreno R, Thisted R. Incidence of postdural puncture headache in morbidly obese parturients. Reg Anesth 1994;19:361–3.
13. Peralta F, Higgins N, Lange E, et al. The relationship of body mass index with the incidence of postdural puncture headache in parturients. Anesth Analg 2015; 121:451–6.
14. Miu M, Paech MJ, Nathan E. The relationship between body mass index and post-dural puncture headache in obstetric patients. Int J Obstet Anesth 2014; 23:371–5.
15. Angle P, Thompson D, Halpern S, et al. Second stage pushing correlates with headache after unintentional dural puncture in parturients. Can J Anaesth 1999;46:861–6.

16. Scavone BM, Wong CA, Sullivan JT, et al. Efficacy of a prophylactic epidural blood patch in preventing postdural puncture headache in parturients after inadvertent dural puncture. Anesthesiology 2004;101:1422–7.

17. Jagannathan DK, Arriaga AF, Elerman KG, et al. Effect of neuraxial technique after inadvertent dural puncture on obstetric outcomes and anesthetic complications. Int J Obstet Anesth 2016;25:23–9.

18. Aida S, Taga K, Yamakura T, et al. Headache after attempted epidural block: the role of intrathecal air. Anesthesiology 1998;88:76–81.

19. Segal S, Arendt KW. A retrospective effectiveness study of loss of resistance to air or saline for identification of the epidural space. Anesth Analg 2010;110: 558–63.

20. Stein MH, Cohen S, Mohiuddin MA, et al. Prophylactic vs therapeutic blood patch for obstetric patients with accidental dural puncture – a randomized controlled trial. Anaesthesia 2014;69:320–6.

21. Al-metwalli RR. Epidural morphine injections for prevention of postdural puncture headache. Anaesthesia 2008;63:847–50.

22. Ayad S, Demian Y, Narouze SN, et al. Subarachnoid catheter placement after wet tap for analgesia in labor: influence on the risk of headache in obstetric patients. Reg Anesth Pain Med 2003;28:512–5.

23. Baysinger CL, Pope JE, Lockhart EM, et al. The management of accidental dural puncture and postdural puncture headache: a North American survey. J Clin Anesth 2011;23:349–60.

24. Baraz R, Collis RE. The management of accidental dural puncture during labour epidural analgesia: a survey of UK practice. Anaesthesia 2005;60:673–9.

25. Gynaydin B, Camgoz N, Karaca G, et al. Survey of Turkish practice evaluating the management of postdural puncture headache in the obstetric population (1). Acta Anaesthesiol Belg 2008;59:7–12.

26. Newman MJ, Cyna AM. Immediate management of inadvertent dural puncture during insertion of a labour epidural: a survey of Australian obstetric anaesthetists. Anaesth Intensive Care 2008;36:96–101.

27. Russell IF. A prospective controlled study of continuous spinal analgesia versus repeat epidural analgesia after accidental dural puncture in labour. Int J Obstet Anesth 2012;21:7–16.

28. Verstraete S, Walters MA, Devroe S, et al. Lower incidence of post-dural puncture headache with spinal catheterization after accidental dural puncture in obstetric patients. Acta Anaesthesiol Scand 2014;58:1233–9.

29. Halker RB, Demaerschalk BM, Wellik KE, et al. Caffeine for the prevention and treatment of postdural puncture headache: debunking the myth. Neurologist 2007;13:323–7.

30. Cohen S, Ramos D, Grubb W, et al. Sphenopalatine ganglion block: a safer alternative to epidural blood patch for postdural puncture headache. Reg Anesth Pain Med 2014;39:563.

31. Kent S, Mehaffey G. Transnasal sphenopalatine ganglion block for the treatment of postdural puncture headache in the ED. Am J Emerg Med 2015;33:1714.e1-2.

32. Gormley JB. Treatment of postspinal headache. Anesthesiology 1960;21:565–6.

33. Riley CA, Spiegel JE. Complications following large-volume epidural blood patches for postdural puncture headache. Lumbar subdural hematoma and arachnoiditis: initial cause or final effect. J Clin Anesth 2009;21:355–9.

34. Paech MJ, Doherty DA, Christmas T, et al, Epidural Blood Patch Trial Group. The volume of blood for epidural blood patch in obstetrics: a randomized, blinded clinical trial. Anesth Analg 2011;113:126–33.

35. Jo D, Kim ED, Oh HJ. Radicular pain followed by epidural blood patch. Pain Med 2014;15:1642–3.
36. Carlswaerd C, Dearvish B, Tunelli J, et al. Chronic adhesive arachnoiditis after repeat epidural blood patch. Int J Obstet Anesth 2015;24:280–3.
37. Devroe S, Van de Velde M, Demaerel P, et al. Spinal subdural haematoma after an epidural blood patch. Int J Obstet Anesth 2015;24:288–9.
38. Hebl JR, Horlocker TT, Chantigian RC, et al. Epidural anesthesia and analgesia are not impaired after dural puncture with or without epidural blood patch. Anesth Analg 1999;89:390–4.
39. Collier CB. Blood patches may cause scarring in the epidural space: two case reports. Int J Obstet Anesth 2011;20:347–51.

Index

Note: Page numbers of article titles are in **boldface** type.

Anesthesiology Clin 35 (2017) 169–180
http://dx.doi.org/10.1016/S1932-2275(16)30107-0
1932-2275/17

anesthesiology.theclinics.com

Moving?

Make sure your subscription moves with you!

To notify us of your new address, find your Clinics Account Number (located on your mailing label above your name), and contact customer service at:

Email: journalscustomerservice-usa@elsevier.com

800-654-2452 (subscribers in the U.S. & Canada)
314-447-8871 (subscribers outside of the U.S. & Canada)

Fax number: 314-447-8029

Elsevier Health Sciences Division
Subscription Customer Service
3251 Riverport Lane
Maryland Heights, MO 63043

To ensure uninterrupted delivery of your subscription, please notify us at least 4 weeks in advance of move.

Printed and bound by CPI Group (UK) Ltd, Croydon, CR0 4YY

08/05/2025

01864696-0007